SUGAR freed

STOP LOSING THE WEIGHT-LOSS BATTLE...

START GAINING THE VICTORY!

CHRISTINE TRIMPE

Praise For SugarFreed: Stop Losing the Weight-Loss Battle, Start Gaining the Victory by Christine Trimpe

As I read Christine Trimpe's vulnerable story, I marveled at how she faithfully points us to the bondage-breaking power of God's redemptive plan in our physical and spiritual lives. Chapter after chapter, I was reminded of Revelation 12:11, which promises how we will one day triumph over our chief enemy, the devil, and experience victory in every sin-struggle and sadness he taunts us with. We're told, "They triumphed over him by the blood of the Lamb and by the word of their testimony." In our final days upon this old earth, the accuser of our souls (who loves to keep us bound up in obesity, lethargy, and self-loathing) will himself be bound up and thrown out of our lives altogether! How? By the saving work of Christ and the testifying word of the saved! That's what will happen then, but it's also how we can battle him here and now, today.

SugarFreed is Christine's testimony of how God set her free, inviting each of us into freedom as well! Only the blood of the Lamb can heal the wounds that food has never been able to. And your testimony holds the power to bring others with you into health and hope! As you consider reading SugarFreed, I encourage you to invite a friend or two to join you on this bondage-breaking journey to freedom!

—**Wendy Speake**, best-selling author of *The 40-Day Sugar Fast* and *The 40-Day Feast*

Christine Trimpe's SugarFreed is a beacon of hope for anyone struggling with weight and health. Your battle with obesity is not entirely your fault, and this book offers practical steps and heartfelt encouragement to address the root cause—insulin resistance. Break free from the hold of sugar and processed carbs once and for all.

—**Jason Fung, MD**, *New York Times* best-selling author of *The Obesity Code*

This book is a testament to the possibility of change and freedom from food addiction. Trimpe's coaching expertise and personal insights make this book a valuable ally for anyone seeking to overcome sugar cravings and obesity.

—**Andreas Eenfeldt, MD**, Founder and CEO,
Diet Doctor and *Hava*

Christine's inspiring, faith-based journey is nothing short of transformational. Her evolution of finding herself, reversing poor metabolic health, and becoming a wellness coach to continue helping others is incredibly motivating. Sugar addiction is the basis of so many diseases and ill health in our current society, and Christine's detailed book will be a well-sought-after resource for patients and clients alike.

—**Cynthia Thurlow, NP**, host of *Everyday Wellness* podcast, 2x TedX speaker, best-selling author of *The Intermittent Fasting Transformation*, passionate advocate for women in perimenopause and beyond

I am very impressed after reading Christine's Sugar*Freed* about her battle with food and weight for many years. I know how hard it is and the pain it bears. The consequences are numerous and so devastating, and behind the battle lies shame and a feeling of failure when dieting, losing weight, relapsing, gaining it back, and more. As you read Sugar*Freed*, you will soon understand why sugar addiction is not your fault. Surrendering to that fact and asking for knowledge and help is your ticket to freedom. I am grateful to Christine for sharing her story and getting a certification in diagnostics and treatment so she can share her deep insights and a new toolbox with others. I know you will be grateful too.

—**Bitten Jonsson, RN, Addiction Specialist ACRPS**;
Founder of *SUGAR® Diagnostic* and *Holistic Medicine
for Addiction Education and Training*

Christine Trimpe's Sugar*Freed* is a powerful guide for anyone struggling with sugar addiction and unhealthy habits. With deep faith and personal insight, Christine walks readers through the essential steps of turning their health around—physically, mentally, and spiritually. From confronting chronic health issues to breaking free from sugar's stronghold, she provides practical advice for lasting transformation. Sugar*Freed* will inspire you to reclaim your health and live in the freedom God desires for you.

—**Susan Neal, RN, MBA, MHS,** author of
7 Steps to Get Off Sugar and Carbohydrates

Eloquent and compelling—Sugar*Freed* tells Christine's story in a way that will speak to your heart and give you the power to look inward at what holds you captive. She is the best friend who has been there and will hold your hand while lifting your chin to the One who breaks every chain.

—**Amanda Decker FNPc, MHP, CKNS,**
@deckerlesscarbs, owner of Clear Path Medical

The apostle Paul wrote, *"For while bodily training is of some value, godliness is of value in every way, as it holds promise for the present life and also for the life to come" (1 Timothy 4:8).* Paul's point is that there are many false teachings that sound like truth, taste like truth, but are indeed not truth. They might give us an emotional boost in the moment, but they do not sustain us.

In many ways, biblical false teaching is like sugar. It can look appealing and taste sweet but doesn't fuel your body. Instead, as sugar makes you a slave to more sugar, false teaching keeps you a slave to sin. You must keep returning to fill your emotional plate because it is incapable of true transformation.

Few people I know understand this as well as Christine Trimpe! Living Sugar*Freed* will cut the chain to the idol of food in your life. The apostle Paul says that healthy living is profitable and valuable. But even greater is godliness. Christine marries these two things wonderfully in this book!

—**Adam Groh,** senior pastor, Berkley Community Church

Seeking true freedom from sugar addiction and unsustainable dieting? Get ready to completely transform your life, mind, body, and soul! By implementing Christine's principles outlined in this book, you can achieve lasting transformation. Sugar*Freed* will unveil God's plan to accomplish infinitely more than you can envision, echoing Paul's words in Ephesians 3:20. Christine's approach to overall wellness and freedom from sugar is truly sustainable. If you're urgently seeking to break the chains of your unhealthy relationship with sugar and experience lasting freedom, SugarFreed is your guide. This book provides scientific facts, practical steps, and spiritual insights to help you realize the freedom you've longed for. SugarFreed is victory waiting to happen for anyone ready to embrace true transformation.

—**Cherie Denna**, award-winning author of *Beloved Outcast: The Quest for True Belonging,* pastor of women's ministry, and founder of the *Everyday Belonging Movement*

Cover design by Amber Weigand-Buckley, Barefaced Creative Media. Front cover photos were provided by Woman's World, Englewood Cliffs, NJ, and photographed by Mary DuPrie Studios, Pontiac, MI, and the author. Author back cover photo by Christina Custodio, Agapeland Photography, Greenville, SC. Restored photo by Sarah Wyatt-Stahl, You and Eye Photography, Berkley, MI. All images are used with permission.

979-8-9887490-2-8 (Paperback)

Library of Congress Control Number: 2024920834

PRINTED IN THE UNITED STATES OF AMERICA

This book is dedicated to the memory of my dear friend of fifty years, Cyndi (Creech) Crossno, a fellow weight-loss warrior and cherished sister in Christ. We stood by each other through thick and thin—literally and figuratively. Cyndi, my heart aches from your early departure, but I celebrate that you've gained the ultimate victory in Jesus. I can't wait to join you in the heavenly realms for a carefree feast with our Savior. Until then, my dear friend, I will serve the Lord boldly, as you exemplified beautifully throughout your life.

Contents

FOREWORD

■　■　■

I am deeply honored to write this foreword for Sugar*Freed*. This book resonates with me on so many levels. As someone who has also faced lifelong struggles with obesity and prediabetes, I found Christine Trimpe's insights both relatable and profoundly enlightening. My personal journey has allowed me to help many patients by sharing my struggles and realizations regarding lifestyle changes. For seventeen years, I felt frustrated by a medical system that did not focus on the root causes of these issues. Christine, however, does an excellent job of applying principles from the Bible to our struggles with sugar addiction, offering a refreshing and holistic perspective.

Recently, I started rucking—carrying a forty-five-pound backpack while hiking. This experience made me realize how much our spiritual and emotional struggles can weigh us down, preventing us from fully pursuing our goals. Struggling under this burdensome extra weight, I had to rest multiple times, moving slowly. But without the rucksack weight, I reached the peak effortlessly. Christine brings this idea to life, discussing how our emotional baggage and spiritual struggles can hold us back. Her grounding in Scripture provides a beacon of hope and direction.

Christine opens the door for the rest of us by sharing her struggles and successes with transparency and courage. Many of us have been held back by strongholds and negative self-talk, unaware of our full potential. This book allows us to rediscover the truth of God's faithfulness and our ability to move forward when life gets challenging. Paul stated in Romans 7:15–17, "*I do not understand what I do. For what I want to do I do not do, but what I hate I do. And if I do what I do not want to do, I agree that the law is good. As it is, it is no longer I myself who do it, but it is sin living in me."*

Many of us know what to do but struggle to follow through. We often give in to temptation and forget our purpose. Christine's outstanding writing provides a clearer vision of what it takes to succeed and the confidence to move forward.

I am thrilled you are starting this journey equipped with the skills and encouragement you'll find here. You can accomplish much more than you currently believe you can. Just take one step. Don't let setbacks deter you from reaching your goals. Never give up on your journey and your desire for health improvements. Christine's Sugar*Freed* book is a valuable guidebook and companion, offering wisdom, encouragement, and practical advice grounded in faith and personal experience.

May this book inspire you as it has me. May you find the strength and determination to break free from the chains of sugar addiction and your weight loss battle to embrace a healthier, more fulfilling life.

With heartfelt encouragement,

Brian Lenzkes, MD

Host of *Life's Best Medicine* and *Low Carb MD* podcasts

INTRODUCTION

SUGAR*FREED* ME

I yearned for freedom my entire life. I craved after *it,* yet my body, mind, and spirit never articulated the exact missing piece of my soul. For almost five decades, the holes, the nooks, the crannies in my shattered heart longed to be filled. But with *what* exactly?

I never could quite put my finger on *it* and *what.* Not really, anyway. But the physical, emotional, and spiritual need for *it* and *what* hovered over my whole being, relentlessly tapping me on the shoulder, grabbing my attention in short bursts, and then quickly slipping out of my hands again. And again. And again.

Can you relate? Can you name the *one* thing that satisfies your entire being—the *it* and the *what* to fill the empty spaces? It took me fifty years to find *it,* and once I did, I couldn't share *it* fast enough.

As my chronic health issues mounted, I felt physically exhausted, emotionally on edge, and spiritually empty, but *it* constantly whispered to me. When I began to find freedom, I documented my new health journey, and as I began to type, my fingers couldn't keep up with the flow of words. I typed as fast as possible, fearing *it* was slipping away from my fingers again. But mostly, because maybe you need this *it* and this *what* in your life, too.

Memories flood my heart. Heartbreaking memories. But also essential memories in my zigzagging journey as I chased the *it* and the *what.* These stories, etched in my soul, longed to burst forth. Memories are not only instrumental but necessary in a healing journey! I had to write them on paper for you as quickly as possible. Especially the one story that catapulted me into a brand-new lifestyle—a way of life that would usher in freedom and satisfy the hunger of my body, mind, and spirit.

I can pinpoint the exact moment when I finally had the resolve to reach up for help from my decades of despair and chronic health issues. My rescuer grabbed me by the wrist and began the hard labor of pulling my desperate self out of the early grave I was heading toward. In my state of morbid obesity, this rescuer had a heavy burden to carry, indeed. But at that moment, I decided to trust. And as I recall and reflect, I realize *this* was the day I discovered the truth that would finally set me *free*.

That's *it*! I finally realized *what* I had been missing in my decades of wandering in a parched desert. It was the lifelong, unfulfilled craving of my body, mind, and spirit. I was craving *freedom* in every aspect of my being, physically and, more importantly, emotionally and spiritually. For decades, I longed to be set *free*—and my very casual approach to my family's faith held me captive for almost fifty years.

That day, I stopped living as a *casual* Christian and began the journey to deepen my relationship with Jesus. He met me in my mess and began breaking the chains of bondage, my *sugar shackles*, link by link, from decades of obesity and addiction to food and sugar. During all those years of wandering while searching for *freedom*, I realized I comforted and filled the aching parts of my soul, those empty spaces in my heart, with something *I thought I could control*—unhealthy food and eating habits. But my habits were way out of control.

What unfolded in my life still feels too good to be true. Jesus grabbed my hand, helped me discover a wholesome and nutritious way to fuel my body and soul, and finally *freed* me from decades of addiction to food and sugar.

Now it's my honor and privilege to share the saving truth I now know. Jesus offers the freedom we need, and He is everything we need to satisfy the hunger of our entire being—body, mind, and spirit.

Living SugarFreed has transformed my whole physical, emotional, and spiritual health. Jesus offers the same satisfaction to you. Friend, I invite you to join me in this heart-transforming and joyful journey to living SugarFreed! Now is the time to stop losing the weight-loss battle and start gaining the victory in your health—once and for all. Your whole health depends on it.

With Joy,

Christine Trimpe

SUGAR® Licensed Practitioner

Certified Health & Wellness Coach and Coffee Cup Counselor

Section 1: Resolving "It"

■ ■ ■

Resolve (verb): to deal with successfully: clear up.[1]

You have *filled my heart* with *greater joy* than
when their grain and new wine abound.
—Psalm 4:7 (NIV), emphasis mine

Chapter 1

Turning "It" Around to Take the First Step

■ ■ ■

Picture this. You find yourself on a majestic mountain trail, surrounded by the breathtaking beauty of God's creation in the crisp, fall, fresh air. At this elevation, with such an awe-inspiring view, your spirit should be elated! Invigorated! Exhilarated! Yet, the reality is different; you are exhausted and exasperated. Gasping the thin air, you realize you can't manage another step. You can't climb. And so, you sit on the sidelines of life … again.

That was me.

Sitting alone on a stump on the side of that mountain trail, tears streaming, my heart longed for freedom and a meaningful life. I no longer wish to sit on a stump alone, so I invite you to take a seat. Settle in with me. It's time to talk—*heart to heart*.

For thirty years, I carried the heavy weight of deep emotional turmoil, craving and comforting myself with all the wrong things. I couldn't climb over any circumstance in my life.

How about you? Are you struggling too? What weight are you trying to carry up this mountain? Friend, I learned you can't climb mountains carrying heavy chains.

"God, I just want to feel better," I mumbled honestly and in humiliation. But in that moment of surrender, something incredible happened. God heard, answered, and led me on a healing journey in my body, mind, and spirit!

And, yes, in this monumental moment of my life, in my state of morbid obesity, I was concerned about my health—but God was about to grab hold of my heart forever.

Think back to a monumental moment in your life—a turning point, a fork in the road, or a life-changing shift in perspective. Some might describe this as an *aha!* or lightbulb moment shining new light in a dark space. We all have them, sooner or later. Have you reached yours yet?

Something, somewhere, *someone*... invites us to step out of the darkness and set aside all our preconceived notions and beliefs. But fear often overpowers and deflects this invitation to step up and step out.

Fear holds us back when we must take a gigantic leap of faith and embrace change. I know this truth because I recently found myself at a crossroads. For thirty years, fear controlled me. The fear of starting and falling flat on my face *again*. The fear of failure. The fear of what others think of me. These fears weighed heavy on my heart and were preventing me from realizing what it means (and what it takes) to live whole and healthy in body, mind, and spirit. Do you feel the heavy weight of fear?

The story of my turning point started as a morbidly obese forty-eight-year-old woman who found herself miserable on her twenty-fifth-anniversary trip. Now, you would think this celebration would fill me with great joy. Instead, I endured the travel while physically suffering various health issues (including an extra one hundred pounds I carried around), being emotionally distant, and spiritually absent from a purpose in life.

As the crisp morning chill lifted, my husband, Rob, and I parked in an overcrowded Rocky Mountain National Park lot. Oh, what a relief to have found a parking spot close to the trailhead as someone departed this early morning. (Thank you, random stranger!) The thought of taking extra steps exhausted me before I had even left the car.

Rob grinned ear to ear over the upcoming events for the day. He had planned for months to explore this park in the mountains of the beautiful state of Colorado. Ah, I love the beauty and the majesty of mountains. The mountain landscape truly beckons my heart and soul. But in the deepest part of my being, I dreaded climbing up a mountain. I craved rest before we had even hit the path.

First, we explored the path around Bear Lake. Gorgeous yellow aspen leaves reflected a jaw-dropping scene of the beauty of God's creativity. Our stroll permeated peace and serenity. I accomplished this hike without breaking a sweat or flaring my knee pain. It was just shy of a mile and not overly strenuous. I convinced myself, "It's a flat walk. I can do flat. I'm a hiker, right?" I thoroughly enjoyed it.

But then, off to the side, stood a post marker for the real hikers. Of course, I appeased my husband to check it out. I contemplated the marked trails, specifically the half-mile trail, to discover Nymph Lake. Rob had planned and wanted to do this hike! A half-mile? Certainly, I possessed the stamina to hike another one-mile round trip. We set off on this trail to find the glassy lake he had read about in park blogs.

I reached my peak. Not *the* peak. I don't mean the pinnacle of this trail. I stopped dead in my tracks halfway up this half-mile incline.

"I'll just wait here, but you go on ahead," I gasped, sucking in air. I moved my bottom to a tree stump that offered a seat to catch my breath.

"Wait, what? Are you sure? I think we are almost at the lake. Not much further. You can do it," Rob encouraged.

I gasped some more. "I'm sorry, I just don't think I can make it on this knee. Plus, I'm out of breath," I mumbled, reasoning that the mountain elevation and thin atmosphere were causing my shortness of breath. "I think I'm experiencing some altitude sickness." Not the first time I've made excuses for my poor health.

"Okay, well, when I get there, I won't stay long," he promised. Rob headed up the path with his back to me.

Dark sunglasses covered my blue eyes. There's no way he or anyone else witnessed the welling tears. I wished to disappear into that stump. A self-defeating, imaginary dialogue tormented my mind:

Look at the obese woman. No wonder she can't make it up this trail, chided Hiker A.

If she had any self-control, she'd not be stuck sitting there like a bump on a log, judged Hiker B.

Maybe she should get up and move her body. She obviously needs more physical activity, shouted Boot Camp Hiker C.

I know, I know, I know…my mind screamed in agreement with them and cut into my soul.

My shattered heart struggled to accept how much and how often I had let my husband down. He had to go alone on his first trip to a beautiful mountain range—disappointment for him, devastation for me.

I whispered, *"God, I just want to feel better."* That's it. That's all I could muster behind my trickle of tears. I was not about to end up sobbing on the side of that trail.

And that, dear friend, is the pivotal moment when I arrived at my breaking point—*my turning point*—a sudden and deep longing for a new path. Deep down, I believed that if I didn't channel this pain and hurt into a positive transformation, I would soon face the point of no return.

It's true. This memory pains my heart and sometimes leaves a little tear in my eye to this day. But the embarrassment of this trip changed my life for the better. By the way, I have a picture of this moment on the stump! You can find a whole scrapbook of photos through the link on the Sugar-*Freed* Resources page at the back of the book.

Believe it or not, there's more to this story.

My poor husband traversed all the trails on his own, but he also had to endure sleepless nights the entire trip because of my obnoxious snoring. Poor man! Unable to smother the noise in our lodgings, Rob kindly informed me that my snoring escalated in the mountain atmosphere. *Oops.* He was unable to escape. *Oops, again.* And I, the snorer, found him shaking me many times during the night, which was extremely annoying and exhausting for us both.

Yes, I reckoned, "It's now or never." So when I got home, I resolved to make severe changes in my life, including scheduling the sleep study I had put off for years. Reflecting on this resolution, little did I know where this newfound resolve would lead.

The Mountains Are Calling

I was born in the Allegany Mountains of Western Pennsylvania. Perhaps that's why mountains ignite my soul. I've always loved the saying, "The mountains are calling, and I must go," from the famous outdoor enthusiast

John Muir. One of the earliest naturalists in United States history, Muir is known as one of the original fathers of the National Park System. He penned this well-known phrase in a letter to his sister in 1873. His complete sentiment goes on to say, " … and I will work on while I can, studying incessantly."[2] Mr. Muir sounds like a determined pioneer, making discoveries to leave a legacy for us all.

As I share my stories with you, I'm channeling Mr. Muir's enthusiastic spirit to pass along. Are you at a crossroads in your health? Do you have a scary health diagnosis calling you to your turning point? Are you gasping for air? At your breaking point? Feeling sick and tired of feeling sick and tired? Are you ready for radical change to impact your life and your whole health—physically, emotionally, and spiritually? Are you willing to try something new?

Friend, this is your moment of truth. I lived with obesity and deteriorating health my entire adult life. And I lived in fear. I was practically afraid of my own shadow as it loomed largely and taunted me with an exaggerated image of myself. Fear paralyzed me in social situations and kept me at home in isolation. I feared being unseen, while on the flip side, I feared being seen! It seems absurd, I know! Have you ever feared walking into a room and being the fattest person there? Do you fear rejection? Does any of this resonate?

All of this left me living in overwhelming guilt and full of shame. But hear my heart, friend. I threw my mountain of fear into the sea. With new strength, I stomped and kicked fear to the curb. By the grace of God, He made good on His promise to give me the power and faith to move a mountain—a feat I never imagined possible after a lifetime of failures and decades of living without hope for good health.

My deepest desire is to pass this strength and hope to you today. Every day, I pray for one person, yes, just one person like you, to grab hold of the inspiration of my weight-loss success story and embark on your joyful journey to health and wellness. It's time to turn the corner, friend. It's time for you to stop losing this battle and start gaining victory!

Through my story and the stories of others I have coached, I pray you'll discover your turning point and find your motivation for success— your resolve! I pray you will discover encouragement and cling to courage.

If I was able to move this impossible mountain, so can you. And I must let you know where I found this source of inspiration, motivation, encouragement, strength, hope, and courage. See those tall mountains over yonder? *Look up*, friends; your help is there.

A song of ascents.
I lift up my eyes to the mountains—
where does my help come from?
My help comes from the Lord,
the Maker of heaven and earth.
—Psalm 121:1–2[3]

Oh, be still my heart. The mountains are calling, and *we* must go. Are you ready to take your first step to turn things around?

Facing My Fifties

My struggles with obesity span my entire life, from my chubby childhood to this day. That's right, friend—I'm fighting this battle for life even though I'm at a healthy weight.

So many thoughts, ideas, and feelings consumed my mind daily before I decided my life had to change. See if you can relate to some of them.

The heavy weight of my heavy weight weighed heavy on my body.

And mind. *Numb.*

And spirit. *Crushed.*

My entire life consisted of going through the motions to get through the day. The goal for the day? Crawl back into bed.

Wake up! Get ready for work—pack lunches. Get the kids out the door.

Commute to work. Work all day—with an afternoon post-lunch slump—commute home.

Grab a quick snooze on the couch to restore energy to make dinner. Or not make dinner. How about some carryout? That sounds so much easier. "Mom is tired, kids. How about McDonald's?" To which they'd exclaim, "Hooray!"

Maybe I'd go to Bible study one night a week but skip it if I was tired. Then, I'd crawl into bed and try to get some rest so I could face the same thing the next day.

Church on Sunday mornings? Often, I hit snooze.

I was living in chronic exhaustion day in and day out. *Complete with brain fog.* I honestly don't know how I functioned mentally day by day.

My spiritual walk was pathetic—*apathetic.*

Overweight by one hundred pounds, my body fat percentage comprised nearly 50% of my weight. These health markers classified me as morbidly obese on my short, five-foot, one-inch frame.

I'll share all the damaging effects of sugar on my health in the section "Restoring Your Body," but trust me—I lived a joyless life.

Deep down in my soul, I knew there had to be a better way. I would attempt, time and time again, the latest and greatest diet advice offered by mankind. You name it, I did it. *Weight Watchers, Medical Weight Loss Clinic, The Weigh Down Workshop*, gym memberships, the cabbage soup diet, *South Beach Diet*, what am I missing? Too many programs to recall. Oh, the big one, the most expensive one—a liquid protein shake diet. I sipped only chocolate and vanilla protein shakes for almost a year under a hospital program supervised by doctors!

I found the most success in this liquid shake program by losing sixty-five pounds; however, it also resulted in the most significant weight-gain rebound. It was expensive, and it failed. It wrecked me. I resigned myself to the fact that I would be obese for the rest of my life.

A funny thing happens when you are inching up on the next significant decade of your life. I'm sure you understand. For example, I did the liquid shake diet when I was thirty-nine, determined to get to a healthy weight by the time I was forty. Most recently, thoughts of turning fifty nagged in my mind. At the age of forty-eight, I weighed my heaviest, even higher than my two pregnancies. One day, I stepped on the scale and saw 230 pounds flashing back at me—soul-crushing. And I was dieting, exercising, and tracking in a weight-loss app! Panic set in as I approached fifty. The number on the scale reminded me again that it was all pointless. And hopeless. *Would I survive my fifties?*

The shock on the scale messed with my mind but didn't bring me to a breaking point. No major wake-up call for 230 pounds? Numb. *Was I made to be fat?* In misery and defeat and too tired to do anything about it, I stuffed those emotions way down with a hefty serving of junk food high in carbohydrates. This scale shock happened shortly before our anniversary trip to Colorado. No wonder I dreaded those mountain trails.

Remember my question, "Have you experienced your turning point?"

That Colorado adventure was my turning point. I swallowed my pride and faced my fears and failures. Enough was enough. No more "Plan B."

When I returned home, I did something I never wanted to do—making the phone call was hard. I scheduled a sleep study to address my chronic snoring, which most certainly contributed to my chronic exhaustion. I had put this off for years because I could barely sleep comfortably in my bed, much less in a strange bed hooked up to dozens of wires. But as I reflect on my journey, I realize this was an essential *first step* out of my comfort zone and put me on a path to change my life.

Are you ready to take that *first step*? When your health is failing, I know. I understand that taking that first step is the hardest. But I'm here to guide you. Here are a few ideas to inspire you to take your first step today:

- Do something. Something is better than nothing.
- Schedule that doctor's appointment.
- Connect with me for accountability.
- Read transformation stories.
- Take baby steps. Take big steps. What suits you uniquely?
- Track changes to motivate you.
- Understand your *why* and *your why*. Yes, that's two *whys*. We'll dive deeper into the *whys* behind your weight-loss goals in chapter 2.
- Be open to trying something new!

Taking hold of this book marks a significant first step. I am rejoicing with you as you begin to reclaim control of your health. I know both your head and your heart are ready for something big. And so, I'll authentically pour out my story from my heart and with vulnerability to encourage you. I will repeatedly remind you of many things, and most significantly, that this is a matter of a *heart transformation*. Your heart is the wellspring of life! Let's start living from the heart.

I don't know about you, but stories inspire me. As I walked this journey, I read daily weight-loss success stories on my favorite low-carb website, *DietDoctor.com*. They've shared my success story several times (see the Resources page). I'm humbled, not only because they selected and shared my story, but by the positive response it received. By the way, I'd love to read your story, so don't be shy—send it to me.

Speaking of *DietDoctor.com*, this is where I found the resources to change my life once and for all. Through my journey, I experienced victory and formulated *The SugarFreed Me Weight-Loss Solution* program to pass along the key to success: *Learn the science, apply the science, and change your life.*

And so, I want to invite you to take the first step to healing and wholeness. In this section, "Resolving *It*," you will do some soul-searching. The following sections will guide you through "Restoring Your Body," "Renewing Your Mind," and "Redeeming Your Spirit."

Maybe you're not sure where your first step might lead you. I understand. Right at this very moment, will you take action? *Keep reading.* I know the struggle seems futile, and you may have abandoned hope. For thirty years, I repeatedly took the first step and repeatedly failed.

That's right—I said thirty years.

Losing weight will take work, perseverance, and commitment—but what's on the other side of winning this battle? *Freedom!* Health. Energy. Restoration. Renewal. Redemption. And joy! Do you crave joy? A deep, soul-satisfying joy? There's an overflowing joy that comes from waiting, crying, depending, praising, and trusting the Lord, as David expressed in one of my favorite psalms:

I waited patiently for the Lord;
He turned to me and heard my cry.
He lifted me out of the slimy pit,
Out of the mud and mire;
He set my feet on a rock
and gave me a firm place to stand.

He put a new song in my mouth,
A hymn of praise to our God.
Many will see and fear the Lord
and put their trust in the Lord.
—Psalm 40:1–3

Are you ready to climb up from the mud and mire? Yes! The most fantastic joy, as I reflect, was that I didn't know how desperately I needed a new song. God heard the deep cries of my hurting heart, and He rescued me most unbelievably. I still pinch myself.

I'm guessing you need some hope. Maybe a little push in the right direction dished up with a lot of inspiration and encouragement.

Come on, let's walk this path together. After all, challenging journeys are always better with friends. We've got lots of work to do, but I'm excited to coach you through this adventure. You can find freedom and greater joy through faith!

Do you believe me that beginning a new *diet* will be filled with great joy? Trust me, it will be as you ditch the old, dreadful dietary dogma and embrace a Sugar*Freed* lifestyle!

Notes to Self

As we end each chapter, I invite you to write notes to reflect on your circumstances. Because, friend, I get it. I can relate to where you are and where you long to be. I'm honored to stand by your side as we face this battle together and strive for victory.

A crucial step in this process is your commitment to action. In my coaching, I call this practice *transform-action*. To transform, we must act. (I will discuss this much more in the next chapter.) At the end of each chapter, I will prompt you to write a few notes—a note to your former self, a note to your future self, and your commitment to a transform-action step. Here is an example from my experience of what you might write.

A Note to Your Former Self: Remember those tears in my eyes on the side of that mountain path? They stung. A familiar sting as I wandered in poor health for thirty years. Little did I know that God would use that painful moment to change my life. Thirty years was a long wait, but my tiny mustard seed of faith delivered remarkable growth in living healthy and whole for God's glory. What a blessing to trust the right path that God finally called me to explore.

A Note to My Future Self: Envision where I long to be. And not even where I long to be but where God calls me. I didn't step into this journey by coincidence. I'll continue to cling daily to the strategies God gives me to regain my best health physically, emotionally, and spiritually. I see more mountains ahead, and I'm ready to climb.

Transform-Action Task: Schedule a sleep study when I return from my Colorado vacation.

Now it's your turn.

A Note to Your Former Self:

A Note to Your Future Self:

Transform-Action Task:

Chapter 2

Reviewing the Past—How Did We End up Here Anyhow?

Who, what, when, where, and why are the essential elements of a good story. The fact that you've picked up this book tells me you long for a good story—but not about me. Nope. This victory story features you!

I'm writing this book because it's time for you to start gaining victory, too. And friend, I love a good transformation story. So how about we begin together right here and now? Let's focus on something essential as you embark on this journey to living Sugar*Freed*.

It's time to answer the question in this chapter title: How did we (you and I) end up here anyhow?

Right off the bat, I love to ask my coaching clients two short questions: "Why?

And *why*?"

That's right; I repeated myself with two *why* questions. Allow me to explain.

When taking back control of our health, the first question is, "*Why* do I want to lose weight? Or *why* do I need to take back control of my health?"

Typically, you can develop a long list of answers to this easier question like:

- I want to feel better.
- I want to climb the stairs without getting out of breath.

- I want to feel comfortable in my jeans.
- I want to feel good about myself for my daughter's wedding.
- I want to have the energy to get through the day.
- I want to stop being afraid every time I go to the doctor.
- I want to live longer and more vitally so my children don't have to care for me and my poor health.
- I want to improve the outcome of a medical diagnosis I just received.
- I want to get off this dieting rollercoaster once and for all.
- I want to serve God to the best of my ability.

You get the idea. Right now, I want you to grab your journal and come up with at least ten reasons you want to regain control of your health.

You probably won't be surprised to learn that the ten reasons I listed above are my top ten answers to my first *why*. And for me, since I was morbidly obese, this would mean losing a significant amount of weight. God knows I was sick and tired of being sick and tired. How about you?

Most importantly, in addition to my turning point when I couldn't climb the mountain, my diagnosis of nonalcoholic fatty liver disease scared the wits out of me, lighting the fire I needed to act. The idea of liver cirrhosis motivated me to move! I'll share more about this health diagnosis in the "Restoring Your Body" section.

The second most important motivator was imagining my future care. While my chronic health diagnoses mounted, my daughter had just entered the College of Nursing at her university. No doubt the burden of care would fall on her eventually, and I didn't want to be her frequent patient because of my poor health. Yes, they say you must do these things for yourself, but I find it a win-win that I would be doing it for myself and for her.

In hindsight, those are two excellent answers to the first *why* question. Did you make your list yet?

Onto the next "*why*" question. This is where the challenging work resides, and we will explore this in greater detail in the sections "Renewing Your Mind" and "Redeeming Your Spirit." But I want to introduce the question now so it can sit in your mind as we go through this journey together. Here are a few questions to ponder. Grab your journal as you feel prompted to respond.

"Why do I find myself in poor health, unable to break free?"

"Why do I fail in all my weight-loss efforts repeatedly?"

"Why do I run to food, sugar, and snacks when I'm uncomfortable?"

"Why do I turn to food when I'm not even hungry?"

"Why do I mindlessly eat?"

"Why am I hiding the evidence of candy bars and fast-food wrappers in the trash can outside?"

"Why do I obsess about where my next meal comes from?"

Well, you get the idea. Those are extremely tough, soul-wrenching, soul-searching questions to answer. Friend, I know how you feel. I know where you are and where you long to be. Let's strategize our battle plan together as we walk out this journey, linked arm in arm. I'm raising a banner over us now—one of solidarity. Hear the rallying cry as we stand under this banner together. You are not alone. I am in your battle unit; better yet, God provides a banner of protection and love over this hard thing He's called us to do—take back control of our health to the glory of God!

I have a blessing from Psalm 20 for you. Grab a piece of paper and some colored pens, and write out this truth to keep in front of you as you march forward in pursuit of victory.

> May he give you the desire of your heart
> and make all your plans succeed.
> *We will shout for joy when you are victorious*
> and will lift up our banners in the name of our God.
> May the LORD grant all your requests.
> —Psalm 20:4–5, emphasis mine

Can you hear it? Can you hear that rallying cry as you stand under the banner of other Christian soldiers worthy of the call in this battle? You are not alone in this endeavor for better health and wellness. We are standing together under the banner of God and making our requests known to Him. May He give you your heart's desire and make all your plans for better health and wellness succeed. I'm already shouting for joy over your victory today!

It's a Matter of Your Heart

Speaking of the desires of your heart...it's time for another journaling exercise. What are the desires of your heart? I never thought to lay these desires down before the Lord for decades. It felt awkward to me. Does this make you squirm?

I never thought God would care deeply about my health and wellness, but for many decades, I also didn't read God's Word daily. Shortly after that Colorado trip, I picked up my Bible every day, and Jesus transformed my life. *He can do the same for you.*

I quickly discovered that God longs for a close relationship with every one of us. He created us uniquely to worship Him and to live for His glory. Just read the verse above again! I'll share plenty more Scriptures as we go through this book so you can taste and see that the Lord is good. He can and will satisfy every longing of your soul to your heart's desire. Join me in picking up your Bible daily and watching Jesus transform your life—physically, emotionally, and spiritually.

And overall, Jesus will change your heart health.

No, I'm not talking about your cardiologist-approved heart health.

I'm talking about the center of your spiritual life. Biblically speaking, the heart is the *wellspring of life* (Proverbs 4:23).

The heart, in biblical language, is the center of the human spirit, from which springs forth emotions, thoughts, motivations, courage, and action.[4] Your heart transformation is the most exciting part of this journey, so lean in. I'll be hammering the characteristics of the heart a lot through every chapter of this book. It's that important! Examining the heart and what flows out of it is a perfect strategy for gaining victory over your poor health.

Check out this roadmap for a heart transformation. I created an easy acronym for you to remember. Write HEART down the side of a piece of paper like this:

H—Handle Your Emotions

E—Examine Your Thoughts

A—Ask for Motivation

R—Run with Courage
T—Take Action

Stop right here and think about this. If we are honest, we know we wound up here because something was not in check deep in our hearts. I'll list the characteristics of the heart again because I want you to memorize the steps in this path: emotions, thoughts, motivations, courage, and action. Could you write it down? Stick it where you will see it every day. Remember to use my HEART acronym above.

And another challenge: memorize this short verse below. It perfectly captures the essence of this *heart*, body, mind, and spiritual transformation journey in our battle with weight, food, and sugar.

> You have *filled my heart* with *greater joy* than
> when their grain and new wine abound.
> —Psalm 4:7, emphasis mine

I read that verse recently with fresh eyes, and my heart skipped a beat. I wanted to discover more about David's song in this psalm, so I researched it.

First, this verse struck me with solid confidence in how the Lord can change our hearts. As people who overly obsess about our weight, food, and sugar, how can God fill our hearts with greater joy than grain and wine? Not only that, but this psalm implies a celebration surrounding a harvest—when grain and new wine abound. We sure do love to celebrate over food, don't we?

I don't know about you, but I'm positive I celebrated food too much and focused on food as a source of happiness and comfort in my circumstances. And I must confess that I never understood or experienced true joy for decades. Can God fill us with greater joy in our hearts than sugar, food, and drink?

Spoiler alert. *Yes.* But it's a marathon, not a sprint, which is why you have this book in your hand, so muster up. We're only just beginning. This is a long haul, and you've only just enlisted. But I know you are battle-ready. Let's prepare ourselves with a brief exploration of the heart transformation. Remember HEART: Handle your *emotions*. Examine your *thoughts*. Ask for *motivation*. Run with *courage*. Take *action*! You must carry these heart characteristics with you as we march forward for your health and wellness.

Handle Your Emotions

Nothing like starting with the most significant battle, huh? As a writer, I'm inclined to look up definitions of even familiar words. Let's start there. Merriam-Webster defines *emotion* as a conscious mental reaction (such as anger or fear) subjectively experienced as a strong feeling usually directed toward a specific object and typically accompanied by physiological and behavioral changes in the body.[5]

The "Renewing Your Mind" section will cover more about emotion, but let me introduce this truth to you now. In my experience, the emotional battle in my weight-loss journey has been the most complex. Again, as the chapter title asks, "How did we end up here anyhow?" is a loaded question. I'm sure you will agree.

Whether fear-based or celebration-based, we are prone to wander to food when confronted with feelings. Can you relate to these responses?

Sad? *We eat in secret shame.*

Angry? *We slam a pint of ice cream.*

Afraid? *We calm ourselves with excess calories.*

Happy? *We convince ourselves that every celebration is better with food!*

Right here and now, we must admit that our first step in gaining victory is acknowledging what we must overcome. I don't know about you, but I carried a ton of emotional baggage in my trunk of feelings. The heaviness of that junk-filled trunk weighed me down significantly for decades. Heavier than the one hundred extra pounds I carried, if I'm honest.

But don't let that scare you—because remember ... this! God can satisfy you with *greater joy* in your heart than the feeling you get from food. Or from the nagging thoughts of food, which brings us to the following characteristic of the heart.

Examine Your Thoughts

Our thoughts are so powerful. To this day, I wrestle with understanding where they come from, so let's look at Merriam-Webster's definition.

A thought is something (such as an opinion or belief) in the mind.[6]

Opinions and beliefs. I've got plenty of those. How about you? Thoughts are essential in this pursuit of freedom. You had to think about picking up this book. You formed an opinion about the subject matter and must've believed this is something you need. Thank you! I have prayed for you and have very positive thoughts and beliefs that God desires you to step boldly into this journey of freedom. He cares, and so do I. What do you think about that?

I never thought that God cared about my state of health. And I also thought I could fix my health on my own. Are you in the habit of thinking you'll improve your health problems all by yourself? Repeatedly? I did for decades. I counted calories and used spreadsheets, thinking I could make it stick this time.

Each time I fell off the wagon of another diet, I formed very negative opinions about myself. What negative thoughts of yourself do you hold in your heart right now?

How about, "I'm a failure. I can never do anything right. I've let down my loved ones once again. I look like a fool." After decades of failure, I finally ingrained the thought in my mind and heart that living fat was my destiny. But deep down, I knew God didn't want that for me. Even though, as I approached fifty, I had almost given up on living a healthy lifestyle, an innate longing to be free from a life of disease gave me a glimmer of hope. One little thought in my mind never went away and pushed me on to trudge through each day.

Think with me, "There has to be a better way." Hold on to that belief. Together, we will watch God change the negative opinions we hold of ourselves as we strive to think about things to change our health for God's glory for good. I love to think about this verse where Paul writes:

> Finally, brothers, whatever is true,
> whatever is noble, whatever is right,

> whatever is pure, whatever is lovely,
> whatever is admirable—
> if anything is excellent or praiseworthy
> —think about such things.
> —Philippians 4:8

True, noble, right, pure, lovely, admirable … those can motivate your heart. Let's move to the next characteristics of your heart transformation.

Ask for Motivation

Motivation is defined as a motivating force, stimulus, or influence.[7] Motivation is vital to walking in freedom in your physical, emotional, and spiritual health. Friend, we need to move forward with that force, stimulus, and influence to light that fire in our belly.

Let's start with influence. As I mentioned earlier, one thing I enjoyed during my weight-loss journey spurred my motivation—an inspiring success story. Now, God has gifted me with a fantastic, joy-filled success story to share with you, and I pray this will influence you to make your heart change and chase after freedom from all the things that weigh you down.

God also instilled a passion in my heart to complete the training to become a *SUGAR® Licensed Practitioner, Certified Health and Wellness Coach,* and *Certified Coffee Cup Counselor* to help you with your motivation. The ultimate reason I share my story and the stories of my coaching clients on these pages is so you can share your story. Get ready for that, friend! You never know what God has in store for your journey.

As far as a stimulus regarding motivation, these stories will keep you moving in the right direction. They will cause you to act (hang on, that's our last characteristic of the heart). Reflecting on the answers to your *why* questions above will also stimulate you to move forward. All the above is your motivating force! Picture me, your coach, with a whistle in my mouth reminding you to march. I know from experience that this journey is not for the faint of heart, so collect your courage. That's the next part of your Sugar*Freed* heart transformation.

Run with Courage

For almost fifty years, I felt weak, the opposite of courageous. I never thought I measured up to man's standards—so why try? Every year, I relied solely upon my power and felt defeated. I never gave a thought to courage. It's no wonder I can recognize a lack of courage as one answer to "How did I end up here anyhow?"

Courage is the mental or moral strength to venture, persevere, and withstand danger, fear, or difficulty.[8]

Often, we lack courage because we want to remain comfortable. Feeling, thinking, or being motivated to sacrifice our comfortable routines is very uncomfortable. Do you have a comfortable habit of running to food? Sugar or salty snacks? What's going on in the comfort of your mind? *Can you be comfortable being uncomfortable?*

That definition convicts me most through the word *fear.* Fear is a powerful force holding us captive to our old, comfortable patterns of behavior that put us in poor health. Fear is a big topic; I'll share more about it in the upcoming chapter, "Conquering Fear." But I draw your attention to fear as you begin this battle. You must be aware of this fear separating you from stepping up with courage in this pursuit to live Sugar*Freed.* Fear does not come from the Lord. Remember, when you are afraid, gaining victory in your healing journey will be more difficult.

Is this going to be hard? I won't sugarcoat this. Absolutely, this will be one of the hardest things you'll ever do in your life.

But you can be courageous. You can persevere. Take a deep breath and gather that courage. Latch on to it for dear life. It's time for the last step in your heart transformation. It's time to act.

Take Action

Remember the very first question I asked you in chapter one—"Have you reached your turning point?" Of course you have or wouldn't be reading these words. You have reached your turning point! Now is the time for action.

And I mean an action that will move you to where you long to be—living whole and healthy once and for all. This is a positive action. We are putting behind the negative and self-defeating actions of our past.

We define our positive action as achieving something, typically in stages, over some time, and with the potential for repetition. An act of will.[9]

Gulp! An act of will. We know God gives us free will. What do we do with this now? So far, we've gained head knowledge from defining the characteristics of the heart, the center of our human spirit. How will you act? You want to accomplish this health and wellness healing once and for all—what action will you take?

Will you be content with doing this in stages? Please *say yes.*

Will you recognize that this only happens over a period of time? Please *be patient.*

Will you adapt to repetition (and simplicity) in your action steps? Please *trust me* (and more importantly, Jesus) when I tell you to act repeatedly in a particular pattern to develop new habits for your health. Throughout this book, I will repeat myself for your benefit—to act (in case you missed it the first time around).

Action is where it's at. It's where you finally make good on your good intentions to take back control of your life. As you examine and explore your emotions, thoughts, motivations, and courage (remember, you are courageous), you will find yourself compelled to take one step closer to victory daily through each action you take.

Imagine! It will spring forth from your heart, and you will experience a transformation in your life.

You will journey from "How did I end up here anyhow?" to "How can I keep going for the rest of my life?" You will be unstoppable when you get your first taste of living Sugar*Freed* in body, mind, and spirit. Wait and see, and then be ready to be a witness.

Before we dive deeper into your body, mind, and spiritual health, I have a critical topic to discuss in the next chapter: "Craving All the Wrong Things." Because right now, you are probably still asking yourself, "How in the world can I quit sugar for good?" And you know there is sugar in everything!

Well, take *heart!* You don't have to give up everything, my friend. Let's taste and see God's good smorgasbord and His design for what we crave. I promise it will fill you with hope.

A Note to Your Former Self:

A Note to Your Future Self:

Transform-Action Task:

CHAPTER 3

CRAVING ALL THE WRONG THINGS

What do you crave? I've given such deep thought and attention to this question throughout my journey. The idea that God created us to crave impacted me so much that it is a significant theme when I coach clients.

I've wrestled with this question for my entire life. Being unable to pinpoint exactly what I longed for, I needed to figure out why I constantly craved potato chips.

So, I'll ask again. What do you crave today? Take a moment to write an answer in your journal. It might seem like such a simple question, but it's complicated when you ponder it. Let me explain in lay terms.

Your physical body might crave salt. Your body needs salt for many reasons, one being to maintain fluid balance and another being proper nerve and muscle function. If you're deficient in sodium, your body will send you signals. Craving salt is a survival mechanism. Recognizing and satisfying what your body is craving is a complicated process. You must be in touch with what's happening in your body to meet those physical needs.

Emotionally, you may be craving food to cope with stress, trauma, loneliness, sadness, or boredom in your life. Comfort food is, as we all know, comforting! Understanding why you reach for food for comfort is very complicated. I am not qualified to address this academically, but I will share much more with you based on my experiences throughout this journey and what I've learned in my sugar addiction training and as a *Certified Health and Wellness Coach*. I've been trying to understand the depth of why we yearn and will explore more in the "Renewing Your Mind" section on emotional health. I don't mean to scare you—gaining freedom in your emotional health will challenge you most on this journey, but it's oh-so worth it! Hang with me—I have some strategies to make it easier.

Let's make it a bit more complicated and throw in our spiritual selves, too. Regarding your health, you must consider your whole self: body, mind, and spirit. You are a complete person with unique physical, emotional, and spiritual needs. Your deepest longings and yearnings are rooted in your soul. How often do you check in with your soul's cravings? Never? "Never" used to be my answer, too.

Now that I've complicated the idea of cravings, I'll ask again: *What do you crave* to satisfy and comfort these yearnings? I'll go out on a limb and guess the answer is food.

Chocolate? Deep-fried Twinkies? Hot fudge cream puffs? Loaded french fries? Pizza and pop? Salt and vinegar potato chips? I absolutely and completely get it. Potato chips were my thing (the saltier, the better). For over three decades, I fought a battle against food and sugar cravings.

Physically, did I need salt? Sometimes.

Emotionally, what was I feeding? *All* the feels.

Spiritually, what was I stuffing into my soul? Now, that was the big question.

This journey forced me to confront each of these tough questions. And my friend, I will do my best to answer them to pass along some hope that you, too, can live Sugar*Freed*.

Take notice: the examples I gave above for "What do you crave?" are very high in carbohydrates. I found myself in a vicious cycle, constantly craving carbs for my *quick fix*. I had no idea that for almost thirty years, my body was responding not only emotionally and spiritually but also physically to my cravings. I physiologically craved carbs, which destroyed my health.

Before we go further, let me define the word craving:

Craving (noun): great or eager desire, yearning.[10]

Yearning is a great way to describe the holes I attempted to fill. I had an infinite number of empty nooks and crannies in my soul—holes in my body, mind, and spirit. I was filling these holes with all the wrong things. How about you?

But stick with me. Put down the pop and the chips and listen up. What if I told you that after years of unsuccessful, hopeless dieting, you could break your vicious cycle? Are you excited to learn an alternative lifestyle that can radically change your life? Your whole life—your physical body, your emotional mind, and your spirit and soul. I hope you're open to the suggestion because the story of defeating my cravings is true. The healing I've experienced can be your story too. Discovering what I craved led me to the victory and freedom I longed for.

I'm so excited to share with you why you are physiologically craving carbs and how ditching carbs and living Sugar*Freed* can improve your health once and for all.

I want to inspire you with my success in applying the science of a sugar-free (low-carb) lifestyle and recommendations of trusted resources.

You'll hear me call this a *lasting lifestyle transformation*. This is not just another diet. Repeat after me. *This is not another joy-sucking, dreadful diet!*

We must be in this for life, and trust me, once you taste this freedom from living whole and healthy, you'll never want to return to your old patterns and behaviors. We won't experience complete transformation and restoration until we reach the other side in heaven. But in the meantime, this work in process (me and you) will resolve daily to heal, restore, renew, and redeem our relationship with sugar and food—through faith!

Above all, I want to share how God began completely flipping my cravings for carbs to solely (or should I say *souly*?) craving His joy. His peace. His goodness. His perfect health plan. I discovered freedom I'd never experienced by ditching sugar and unhealthy carbs. God and God alone can satisfy the hunger of body, mind, and spirit through this journey with Him. Remember Psalm 4:7 about the heart? This is a key verse in my life. God can fill you with freedom and greater joy than any food or drink. It's true.

As I mentioned, my despair increased as I approached each new decade in life. The countdown clock quickly ticked to another milestone birthday—fifty. And I was still sick, still fat, and still exhausted.

My body constantly craved carbs, my mind was soothing itself with carbs, and my spirit neglected the one trustworthy source of hope. Truly, God was my only hope and source of strength to break this cycle of fueling myself with carbs. I was neglecting God's interest in my health, which was reflected, in the physical sense, through a lifestyle of dependence on a high-carb, Standard American Diet (SAD).

But you see, I needed to understand why I craved carbs physiologically. There is a fantastic explanation that no healthcare provider ever shared with me. Let me explain why we crave carbs every day physiologically (defined as a characteristic of or appropriate to an organism's healthy or normal functioning[11]).

Let's go back to when I arrived home from Colorado and scheduled the sleep study. If you recall from my turning point story, my obstructive sleep apnea diagnosis led me to research hormones. I learned that adequate sleep is essential to hormone health.

Shortly after that Colorado trip, I also began having extreme abdominal pain. An ultrasound revealed that ovarian cysts were the source of the pain. And surprisingly, I was also diagnosed with fatty liver disease (NAFLD—nonalcoholic fatty liver disease)! I was barely familiar with fatty liver disease, but it sounded scary, so I began my research. This research led me down many rabbit holes, but the most important lesson that I discovered was that sugar is a significant hormone disruptor and a likely culprit to my many health ailments.

What a wake-up call! Sugar. Hmmm. *There's sugar in everything!*

I needed a major lifestyle change if I wanted my health to improve. How about you? Is the way you feel today about your health or chronic issues a major wake-up call? Have you ever considered how much sugar is in the food you consume every day?

After a few months of self-pity, I began to heal my fatty liver and lose the excess weight. I started what I now call my Sugar*Freed* lifestyle, my quitting sugar journey. My first choice? I quit flavored coffee creamer and coffee as the first step in my food choices. You read that right. I quit coffee cold turkey. Talk about a drastic choice! But I had to go big because I never enjoyed black coffee.

Every few days, I picked a new sugar or refined carbohydrate food to give up. Start thinking right now, "What will my first choice be?"

Within a few months, I was ultimately off sugar and refined carbs (factory-processed foods). And by sugar, I mean the sweet stuff, like candy, pastries, and desserts. Sweet treats.

I experienced many positive health improvements, like no more headaches or acne. My daily energy increased between the CPAP machine for my obstructive sleep apnea and the new SugarFreed way of eating.

Most interestingly, my cravings for sugar-filled foods also significantly decreased. Overall, I experienced positive results every day.

However, over ten months, although I adhered strictly to this moderate SugarFreed lifestyle by ditching the sweet white stuff, my body only shed eighteen pounds. Less than two pounds a month; this lack of weight-loss progress worried me about my liver and prediabetes. Do you know how frustrating it is to have brief moments of success and hope and then continuously fail in the quest for permanent weight loss and health improvement? I suspect you know the frustration I experienced because I'm guessing you have experienced it, too. It's like a longing in the heart mentioned in this proverb:

> Hope deferred makes the heart sick,
> but a longing fulfilled is a tree of life.
> —Proverbs 13:12

I see that longing in your heart. I understand the reason you're craving carbs. I have walked in your shoes. I also experienced deferred hope. But I have good news.

What if I told you this is not all your fault? Would you believe me? I'm just a gal busting at the seams to tell you how I lost over one hundred pounds and will never be obese again.

My success may inspire you, but I'm not a scientist or a doctor. How can I confidently tell you this? I have a trusted source I will share with you. This source was the key to defeating my lifetime of being stuck in obesity while facing mounting health issues. It was truly divine intervention when I stumbled on this source of life-changing information.

On January 13, 2017, I had lunch with a friend. Now, this friend loved to talk about hormones. She spoke to me about hormones for years, and I never paid attention before because I didn't realize I had so many hormonal problems. I complained to her about my slow weight loss despite quitting the white sugar, and she started talking about hormones again. This time, I listened because I knew I needed to fix my hormones.

My friend asked me the question that would radically change my life.

"Have you ever heard about intermittent fasting? This doctor in Toronto talks about fasting and hormones, and you should read his book."

Later that evening, unfamiliar with this doctor or intermittent fasting, I went straight to Dr. Google and googled "hormones and fasting."

Tears still well in my eyes reflecting on this day. It was the day I learned: *Obesity is not entirely my fault; obesity is not wholly your fault.* We have been given poor dietary advice for our damaged metabolism for years. Dr. Google led me to the real-life doctor my friend mentioned, who freely shared the secret to defeating obesity and related chronic health issues for people like me. People like you. I cried as I read his words and watched his videos, where he told me, "This is not your fault." Jason Fung, MD, a nephrologist in Toronto, Canada, explained this life-changing information to me:

> The real problem is the acceptance of the underlying assumption that obesity is all about "Calories In, Calories Out." This failed CICO mentality has pervaded our entire universe, and the natural conclusion of this line of thinking is that if you are obese, "It's your fault that you 'let yourself go.'" You either failed to control your eating (low willpower, gluttony) or did not exercise enough (laziness, sloth). But it is not true. Obesity, as I've written about in *The Obesity Code*, is not a disorder of too many calories. It's a hormonal imbalance of hyperinsulinemia. Cutting calories when the problem is insulin is not going to work. And guess what? It doesn't.
>
> Not only do people with weight problems suffer all the physical health issues—type 2 diabetes, joint problems, etc., but they also get blamed for it. Blame that is unfairly targeted toward them because the advice they received to lose weight had a 99% failure rate. Should people get angry about it? Absolutely.[12]

Unbelievable. I'd been told for years that I had *insulin resistance* (another term for hyperinsulinemia that Dr. Fung references above), but not one healthcare provider explained it to me as Dr. Fung did through a random Google search! "Blame that is unfairly targeted toward them…" May I finally be able to release my guilt and shame over my lifetime of obesity? We will explore guilt and shame in depth when we get to the chapters on emotional healing. But for now, what are your thoughts on learning obesity is not entirely your fault?

As I mentioned before, I felt awful, so I cried out to God for healing as my health problems mounted. Emotions overwhelmed me as I listened to Dr. Fung explain that this was not my fault. His practical advice lifted such heaviness from my whole being and provided a unique approach to weight loss for someone like me. And probably someone like you. No doctor or nutritionist had given me such hope in just a few minutes. But I knew this was the path God put right before me. Could this be the answer to my deepest prayers for healing? I decided then and there to jump in with both feet into a new lifestyle incorporating fasting and Dr. Fung's other recommendation of a low-carb diet, which I call the SugarFreed lifestyle!

Dr. Fung's videos and blogs made perfect sense for someone like me, someone who has been suffering from insulin resistance and severely messed up hormones for decades. Not to mention, he explained the science quickly for non-scientific people to understand. (Please, after finishing this book, read *The Obesity Code: Unlocking the Secrets of Weight Loss* by Jason Fung, MD.)

Now armed with the knowledge that my obesity was not entirely my fault, I was empowered to take action. It was not entirely my fault, but it was entirely *my problem*. What I learned from Dr. Fung miraculously worked for me, changing my health and wellness forever. It will work for you, too, if you're ready to act and defeat your obesity problem.

I'll share a condensed version of Dr. Fung's life-changing advice. I knew it would work for me from day one. It very quickly answers the question "What do you crave?" from a physiological perspective. Wouldn't it be life-changing to know why you crave carbs every day?

In the very first video I watched, Dr. Fung explained fasting.[13] His suggestion that fasting could be done for spiritual and health reasons immediately caught my interest. I desperately needed this practice in both areas of my life.

In the video, he explains the role of the insulin hormone as our fat-storing hormone. This brief video made perfect sense and confirmed that I needed to reduce carbohydrates to begin the process of restoring my health. I readily recognized an attribute of my damaged metabolism. I am *carbohydrate-intolerant*. Most overweight individuals are. I'll explain more in the section Restoring Your Body, but here, I want to explain why we crave all the wrong things physiologically.

That evening, while binge-watching Dr. Fung's videos, I determined that intermittent fasting and his suggestion of a low-carb, Sugar*Freed* way of eating could be implemented into my life to improve my health and enable me to lean harder on God. I resolved that I must quit the crazy carb rollercoaster because I realized what insulin hormone imbalance was doing to my health and why it drove me to want to eat constantly.

Let me explain this in the simplest way I can—picture roller coaster tracks. As an insulin-resistant person, if you connected my day's blood sugar test results on a graph, you would see definite spikes with each mealtime. The pattern would look like a wild rollercoaster ride—up and down, up and down. There is a strong correlation between blood glucose results and the insulin response in your body.

First, let me define my former diet and food choices as a high-carbo-hydrate (SAD) diet. My meals typically included scant low-carb options: a little protein, some vegetables, and possibly some cheese. But I mainly filled up on high-carb starches like potatoes, pasta, and bread. And if I had an occasional piece of fruit, it was also very high in sugar. Bananas were my go-to (one medium banana has twenty-seven grams of carbohydrates). To compare my former way of eating, one banana is more carbs than I eat in a day in my Sugar*Freed* lifestyle. Sugar fueled my days every day for almost fifty years.

Back to the rollercoaster ride. Each time I ate a high carbohydrate meal, my insulin and blood sugar would spike. Within an hour, insulin and blood sugar began to decline. Within two hours, the result would be back to the pre-meal levels. This descent is what I call "the crash." As a sugar burner, I experienced a crash after each meal. Have you felt this crash? You may feel like you need a nap. At the bottom of the crash, your body starts *screaming* at you to feed it again. I remember those *"hangry"* days so vividly.

What a vicious cycle—one that is never broken and never gives your body a chance to burn fat for fuel. Each time I ate one of those recommended five to six meals daily, all I burned was sugar (glucose) for fuel. My body never needed to tap into the fat stores because of the excess sugar for energy in my body. And yes, my friend, the staples in my diet (potatoes, pasta, and bread) are very high in sugar. So is popcorn and many other foods. When these starchy foods hit your digestive system, it doesn't know the difference between bread or a slice of chocolate cake. Don't shoot the messenger, please! Keep reading.

Dr. Fung taught me how to get off this crazy insulin spiking, blood sugar surging and crashing, wild rollercoaster ride.

I'm not crazy, friends. There is a physiological reason we crave carbs all day, every day. Why are we just learning about this? Not one healthcare provider shared this with me in thirty years of dieting.

My immediate goal and plan for victory? I implemented Dr. Fung's tools to stabilize my insulin and blood sugar. The new graph you can picture is a relatively flat line. No more spikes. No more crashes. If Dr. Fung is correct, I could anticipate remarkable improvements in my health—and I did! Friend, we now have a method to unlock the secrets of obesity and control our fat-storing hormone: insulin.

And please understand—for the insulin-resistant, carb-intolerant, or those suffering from metabolic syndrome, *weight loss is all about hormones! Again, insulin is our fat-storing hormone.*

It stuns me still that with the knowledge gleaned from one short five-minute video from Dr. Fung, I learned the key to breaking the chains of my lifelong battle with obesity. A true miracle and gift from God. A tool to deal with my flesh, body, and brain cravings.

Breaking the chains of carb addiction led to freedom from food addiction, too. I now had *freedom* from eating a meal I never hungered for in the first place—breakfast. Stopping breakfast ushered in my first *taste of freedom* surrounding food, cravings, and dietary advice that had failed me for many years. I consumed breakfast even when I wasn't hungry because, for decades, people instructed me to eat five to six small meals a day to keep my metabolism active! This was horrible advice for me. All it was doing was fueling my days with glucose and impeding the process of burning fat. So, I stopped eating breakfast and was on my way to my weight-loss dreams.

This brings me back to the important tip I shared earlier: *You must learn the science and apply the science to change your life!* I'm delighted to be your guide, but you and you alone will accomplish this for your health. Remember, *action* will be critical to your success.

Spend time reading (books like this), researching, watching video lectures, and listening to podcasts (check out the Resources page for my guest appearances). There is a plethora of low-carb and Sugar*Freed* advice at our fingertips. If you follow me through social media or my blog, you will find me sharing my favorite resources often. Plus, I have *The* Sugar*Freed Me Weight-Loss Solution* program designed specifically for you. I will share what works for me in the next section, "Restoring Your Body."

Through this research, you will do yourself a tremendous favor in discovering why your years of obesity and chronic health issues *are not entirely your fault!* You are craving sugar and carbs for a reason—a reason you can flip on its head. Doesn't that fill your heart with so much hope? You can live Sugar*Freed*! And the low-carb and fasting lifestyle makes it much easier to walk in this victory once and for all.

I will never be able to express my gratitude for the life-changing information shared by Dr. Fung and *DietDoctor.com*. My best response is to pass this knowledge and valuable resources on to you with real-life stories for inspiration. First, you will experience a new sense of control over your cravings physiologically, which will in turn help you control your emotional and spiritual cravings.

Now that you realize your obesity and chronic health issues are not entirely your fault, I'll share my best Sugar*Freed*, low-carb, and fasting lifestyle tips throughout the rest of this journey—tips for success. Let's start learning the lifestyle to restore your body, renew your mind, and redeem your spiritual walk. You're on your way to my favorite exhortation:

Crave well, choose well—to live and to serve well. All for the glory of God!

A Note to Your Former Self:

A Note to Your Future Self:

Transform-Action Task:

Section 2: Restoring Your Body

■ ■ ■

Restore: (verb) to bring back to or put back
into a former or original state.[14]

Therefore, I urge you,
brothers, in view of God's mercy,
to offer your bodies
as living sacrifices,
holy and pleasing to God—
this is your spiritual act of worship.
—Romans 12:1

Chapter 4

Confronting Chronic

Health Issues

By now, you know that sugar is like a slow poison, leading to chronic health issues. But don't lose hope. Living a Sugar*Freed* lifestyle can reverse and resolve many of the health challenges you face today.

Now, I know what you may be thinking. "Christine, I don't have trouble with sugar. My struggle is with x, y, or z." Let me share a conversation I had in the breakroom with a nurse practitioner after she noticed my dramatic weight-loss success.

"Wow, you are doing amazing with your weight loss! What are you doing?" she asked.

"I quit sugar!"

"Wow? My problem is not with sugar. My problem is potatoes and salty junk food."

"Oh. I hate to break this to you, but potatoes and salty junk foods break down into sugar during digestion. By saying I quit sugar, I mean I quit a diet high in carbohydrates—sweet or savory."

Her jaw dropped. You might think, "How can a nurse practitioner not know this?" Well, in her defense, unless a healthcare provider specializes in obesity medicine, they receive minimal training in nutrition. I didn't know that potatoes and whole wheat bread kept me insulin-resistant for decades. So, I give her a pass. Don't expect your average healthcare provider to understand or explain anything about what's keeping you fat. But again,

I refer you back to hope. Let's find our hope for healing by digging a little deeper into our sugar-filled diet.

Each of us needs to answer the question: *Am I addicted to sugar?* Here are five questions to ask yourself. And be honest. Even if you respond *yes* to one of them, you're most likely addicted to sugar. Keep the word *cravings* in mind. You might find it helpful to grab your journal and record your responses on paper. You'll be glad to have your answers when you share your future victories. And don't forget carbohydrates are sugar.

1. Do you believe a decline in your physical health, such as chronic exhaustion and weight gain, could be linked to sugar consumption? Or the inability to lose weight despite sticking to your daily calorie allowance?
2. Are you full of guilt and shame after overconsuming sugary junk foods and drinks? Do you regret these actions time and time again?
3. Do you hide or lie about your food and sugar habits to those people in your life who are concerned about your health?
4. Have you found yourself consuming larger amounts of sugar to satisfy intense cravings or experience pleasure?
5. When you have tried to reduce your sugar intake, do you experience withdrawal-like symptoms such as irritability, mood swings, or headaches?

The day before I stepped into my quitting sugar journey, my answer to each of these questions was a regrettable *yes*.

Yes, I know my mounting chronic health issues were related to my way of eating a diet high in refined carbohydrates, even if I wasn't binge-eating rows of Oreos. I loved my potatoes, bread, and pasta. And yes, the occasional sugary dessert!

Yes, I felt the weight of guilt and shame every time I overindulged.

Yes, I could easily hit the drive-thru lane for some hot fries to satisfy a craving. The trash can in my garage quickly hid the evidence.

Yes, I recall the days of my savory and sugary vicious cycle of eating. Can you relate to eating something salty, needing something sweet, and then needing something salty—and so on until you're overstuffed?

Yes, I recall mood swings in my attempts to clean up my diet. My poor family!

Again and again, I confess … cravings ruled my life. For decades, I satisfied those cravings with sugar and junk foods, which led to my poor health.

Unsure this is you? Take time to review the questions posed above. Seriously. Is it time to face reality and join me in this time of confession? *Yes*, I am a sugar addict. You may hear sugar and food addiction terminology used interchangeably, so I want to share with you some additional signs of food addiction (the italicized responses are my personal experiences).

1. **Loss of Control.** *Repeatedly eating throughout the day, even when I was not physically hungry. In my mind, the dietary advice to eat 5–6 meals a day fueled this pattern.*

2. **Intense Cravings.** *My thoughts were often obsessive about food, especially foods high in carbs, sugar, and salt.*

3. **Emotional Eating.** *I often turned to food as a source of comfort from stress and boredom and even times of celebration as a reward.* (Note: I'll share more about this in the section "Renewing Your Mind.")

4. **Repeated Patterns Despite Physical Pain.** *I often ate to the point of physical discomfort: tight clothing, acid reflux, bloated stomach, and constipation.*

5. **Fixation on Food.** *This was incredibly disruptive in my life while traveling or finding ways to dine in restaurants. Instead of enjoying conversations with friends and family, I was strategizing where to find the next best meal.*

6. **Failed Attempts in Successful Weight Maintenance.** *Unaware of the impact of carbs and sugar on my insulin hormone, I experienced relapses and returned to unhealthy behaviors due to the addictive nature of carbs for three decades.*

7. **Social Avoidance.** *Shame and embarrassment kept me home more often than not. When I did step into a social event, I always planned to get out, especially at events featuring food.*

8. **Neglect of Responsibilities.** *I always lacked the energy to keep up with household chores.*

9. **Health Consequences in Body, Mind, and Spirit.** *I experienced adverse physical effects, such as obesity, as well as emotional distress, low self-esteem, isolation, and spiritual apathy. I never believed God created me uniquely with a purpose, so why bother?*

Now is the perfect time for you, my friend, to join me in gaining your victory over this stronghold of sugar and junk food and experiencing the weight-loss success you've always imagined! Dream big with me. Join me in the resolve and the action I took next.

I stayed true to my resolve to schedule a sleep study after the Colorado trip. When I called, I asked for an appointment immediately, leaving no option to back out.

Before I run through the gamut of my chronic health issues, I confess that being obese did not spark joy in my life. Quite the opposite. It made me a cranky couch potato. Not to mention, I had some aches, pains, or complaints every day.

Now that you know I am a recovering sugar and food addict, I think setting aside this chapter here is essential to share a bit about my health diagnoses. Not from a clinical approach; I am not a clinician. But what I am is a personal researcher. And a learner. And I'm an upholder. Meaning as I learned I took action, and as a result, I changed my life. You can do the same. Remember my catchphrase:

Learn the science, apply the science, and change your life.

Let's start by discussing my challenges in lay terms and then reading about some of the women I've coached in recent years. They all had chronic health issues and were set free by adopting the Sugar*Freed* lifestyle. I hope my story and theirs will inspire you to act.

———

Christine Trimpe—How Healthy Conviction Changed My Life

My body was a ticking timebomb, a metabolic mess. I rushed toward a life of chronic health issues. I endured daily headaches, monthly migraines, painful periods, joint pain, acid reflux, cystic acne, skin-picking, and chronic exhaustion for decades, not to mention my self-diagnosed mild depression with anxiety and mood disorder. I experienced no joy in any of that.

An onlooker might have described me as happy because that was my public persona. However, now that I know the difference between happiness and joy, I am grateful to choose joy.

Over my years in the various diet programs, doctors diagnosed me with prediabetes, insulin resistance, metabolic syndrome, hyperinsulinemia, ovarian cysts, fatty liver, joint inflammation (heading toward a knee replacement), and obstructive sleep apnea. Polycystic ovarian syndrome (PCOS) wasn't a thing when I was experiencing all the symptoms beginning in my teen years. Considering my years of suffering from debilitating menstrual cycles, I'm sure that PCOS would be added to this list. I also suffered daily from burning acid reflux and monthly outbreaks of cystic acne on my chin that I relentlessly picked at.

Considering all the above, I raced toward an official diagnosis of type 2 diabetes, accompanied by all the horrible potential side effects. Praise God, He intervened in the nick of time. Not one single doctor or nutritionist in all those diet programs shared the full scoop on the dramatic complications of type 2 diabetes—heart disease, stroke, high blood pressure, neuropathy, dialysis, and limb amputation. Wow! I think I'll pass.

Here are the highlights of my metabolic mess.

First and most obviously, *obesity.*

Obesity is a medical condition. Excess body fat accumulates and harms your health. Doctors like to measure obesity with BMI (body mass index). I recall the shameful moment a doctor first told me I was *morbidly obese.* I was mortified and squirmed in my exam gown with nowhere to hide.

A healthy BMI for someone my age and size is between 18.5 and 24.9. A healthy weight range for me would be 100–134 pounds.[15] At my highest weight of 230 pounds, my BMI was 42.7.[16] That's not where my story ends, so stick around, and I'll share my results later.

The word *obesity* never rolled easily off my tongue. I could acknowledge I was fat or overweight but never considered myself *obese.* I never wanted to be there. But there I was, forty-eight years old and not just obese, but *morbidly obese* (a BMI of over 40). Morbidly means, yes, I was on a fast track to a shortened life expectancy.

Obesity leads to *chronic exhaustion.*

This was one of my biggest battles. Exhaustion is a soul-sucker. All I wanted to do was sleep. I took naps often. My kids knew better than to bother Mom when she was napping (this is how I earned my nickname *Crabby Patty*).

I carried around over one hundred extra pounds on my petite frame. That would make anyone tired. Try this: go to the grocery store, grab ten ten-pound sacks of potatoes, and carry those around all at once. I can't even imagine. Living for decades so weighted down—it's mind-blowing.

I suspected the Standard American Diet (SAD) diet caused my sad afternoon slumps. What I didn't know, and what I never checked, was my wild-swinging blood sugar. As I've explained, these blood sugar swings were a primary culprit in my tired existence.

Living tired all the time limited my ability to be active and do fun things with my kids. I sat over on the sidelines, far away from all the action. It broke my heart and crushed my spirit.

Another contributor to exhaustion: *obstructive sleep apnea (OSA).*

I've told you about my obnoxious snoring. Do you know who is a saint? My husband, that's who. My sleep apnea was diagnosed as *obstructive sleep apnea*, not to be confused with *central sleep apnea*. Something obstructed my airway. It was my fat neck. Lowering your body weight has the potential to reverse *OSA.* I had a weight threshold when *OSA* would kick in. From our recollection, anytime I weighed over 180 pounds, we would all get less sleep. Translation: the better part of the three decades of my obese life.

I'm not quite sure why I put off the sleep study for so many years; probably because I had only heard the CPAP machine is uncomfortable to wear at night. Well, sure enough, I was diagnosed with severe *OSA* and sent home with my very own CPAP machine (CPAP stands for *continuous positive airway pressure*). The machine helped me breathe and sleep better again, thank God.

I am grateful I did the sleep study. It is the first step to victory in my lifelong weight-loss battle. When I brought home the CPAP, I used the machine faithfully every night. Both my husband and I immediately benefited from improved sleep.

This is key to my story—*listen up*. Researching *OSA* introduced me to the fascinating world of hormones and their role in our metabolic functioning. It was just enough information to get me thinking about hormones and a precursor to the life-changing knowledge I would gain when I discovered the benefits of quitting sugar for my whole health.

I thought dragging the machine around when I traveled with friends and family would be embarrassing, but the improvement in sleep far outweighed any emotional baggage caused by *OSA*. Sleeping better left me feeling better, and it wouldn't be long before I took the next step in this climb to better health. My spirit stirred in this healing process; I didn't realize how significant this would be then.

I knew nothing about this next health issue: *metabolic syndrome*.

I first heard this diagnosis as a patient in the weight-loss clinic of my local hospital. I asked the doctor to explain *metabolic syndrome* as it was new. Let's check out the definition from the National Institutes of Health:

> *Metabolic syndrome* is a group of conditions that together raise your risk of coronary heart disease, diabetes, and other serious health problems. Metabolic syndrome is also called insulin resistance syndrome.[17]

My doctor advised me I was at risk of all the above and shared a chart with me that included these risk factors, also found on the National Institutes of Health site:

> You may have metabolic syndrome if you have three or more of the following conditions. The five conditions described below are metabolic risk factors. You can have any one of these risk factors by itself, but they tend to occur together. You must have at least three metabolic risk factors to be diagnosed with metabolic syndrome.
>
> - *A large waistline*: This is also called abdominal obesity or "having an apple shape." Extra fat in your stomach area is a bigger risk factor for heart disease than extra fat in other parts of your body.

- *High blood pressure:* If your blood pressure rises and stays high for a long time, it can damage your heart and blood vessels. High blood pressure can also cause plaque, a waxy substance, to build up in your arteries. Plaque can cause heart and blood vessel diseases such as heart attack or stroke.
- *High blood sugar:* This can damage your blood vessels and raise your risk of getting blood clots. Blood clots can cause heart and blood vessel diseases.
- *High blood triglycerides:* Triglycerides are a type of fat found in your blood. High levels of triglycerides can raise your levels of LDL cholesterol, sometimes called bad cholesterol. This raises your risk of heart disease.
- *Low HDL cholesterol, sometimes called "good cholesterol":* Blood cholesterol levels are important for heart health. "Good" HDL cholesterol can help remove "bad" LDL cholesterol from your blood vessels. "Bad" LDL cholesterol can cause plaque buildup in your blood vessels.[18]

I checked off large waistline, known as central obesity, high triglycerides, high fasting blood sugar, and low HDL. Unfortunately, the doctors told me the diagnosis but didn't tell me the why or the impending health crises. In my thirty years of dieting, there was no mention of my fasting insulin hormone nor what that means to an obese person. Time and time again, I was chastised to lose weight, eat less, and move more … yada, yada, yada. If I had known then what I know now, those doctors would be sitting in my lecture. Ha! Sadly, I was too ashamed to address the situation further with the doctors. Sigh.

Metabolic syndrome is also known as *insulin resistance (IR)*. Some doctors will call this *prediabetes*. Doctors diagnosed me as prediabetic for many years. But never once did the doctors use the term *insulin resistant*. What is it? The National Institutes for Health has a great description of *IR / Prediabetes*:

Insulin resistance is when cells in your muscles, fat, and liver don't respond well to insulin and can't easily take up glucose from your blood. As a result, your pancreas makes more insulin to help glucose enter your cells. As long as your pancreas can make enough insulin to overcome your cells' weak response to insulin, your blood glucose levels will stay in the healthy range.

Prediabetes means your blood glucose levels are higher than normal but not high enough to be diagnosed as diabetes. Prediabetes usually occurs in people who already have some insulin resistance or whose beta cells in the pancreas aren't making enough insulin to keep blood glucose in the normal range. Without enough insulin, extra glucose stays in your bloodstream rather than entering your cells. Over time, you could develop type 2 diabetes.[19]

Another term doctors diagnose is *hyperinsulinemia.* I don't recall hearing this term from one of my doctors, but in my research, I discovered it fits my health history, too. Here's an explanation from the National Institutes of Health:

Hyperinsulinemia: Dysregulated insulin secretion and/or clearance resulting in chronically elevated insulin without hypoglycemia is common in obesity and metabolic disorders, and it is referred to herein as hyperinsulinemia. Fasting insulin rises from normal glucose tolerance to impaired glucose tolerance (IGT) to T2D (type 2 diabetes).[20]

For over a decade, I was told by my well-meaning doctors I was *prediabetic,* but not one of them told me why (again). The elephant in the exam room was always my obesity. If only a doctor had explained how insulin worked (or, in my case, didn't work) in my obese body, I could have turned my health around sooner.

"Doctor, I swear I am eating less and moving more! Nothing. Is. Working. Why not?" I knew I was one high blood sugar test result away from being prescribed type 2 diabetes medications. Fear of a future of drug dependency consumed my mind. I never enjoyed living in fear, and now I know God didn't give me a spirit of fear.

One last big surprise: *fatty liver disease (NAFLD)*. In December 2015, I received a diagnosis of NAFLD. The complete medical term for this is *nonalcoholic fatty liver disease*. After years of obesity, it should not have been a surprise that my liver was full of fat, but once again—I had no idea this was even a thing. *My liver was full of fat!* Shouldn't these organs know enough to keep the fat out? Nope.

This diagnosis truly frightened me.

It was time to start evaluating my lifestyle. Left untreated, NAFLD may progress to NASH (nonalcoholic steatohepatitis—a fatty liver with inflammation and cell damage), which may further progress to *cirrhosis of the liver* (an irreversible condition where the liver is scarred and permanently damaged, leading to liver failure). Here are the symptoms and causes of NAFLD and NASH from the National Institutes of Health:

> Usually, nonalcoholic fatty liver disease (NAFLD) is a silent disease with few or no symptoms. Certain health conditions and diseases—including obesity, metabolic syndrome, and type 2 diabetes—make you more likely to develop NAFLD. [21]

Did you catch that phrase? NAFLD has few or no symptoms. In the fall of 2015, when I discovered this, I had no idea that my liver was sick.

My doctor ordered ultrasound scans because I also experienced painful ovarian cysts, which led to the discovery of my NAFLD. Those painful cysts saved my liver. If it hadn't been for those cysts, I wouldn't have started researching NAFLD, and I wouldn't have gone down the rabbit hole of researching how and why this happened and my treatment options.

All my research about NAFLD alerted me to the poison in my diet—*SUGAR!* What could I do about this? *There is sugar in everything*, or so I thought. The more I researched, the more precise the answer became to me. I needed to eliminate sugar from my diet. *Completely.* Lots to ponder. Quitting sugar seemed like an impossible lifestyle change considering the dietary guidelines recommended by the government and all my doctors and healthcare providers.

———

Phew! Those were my messy metabolic health issues—I think it's quite the list! Obesity, chronic exhaustion, obstructive sleep apnea, metabolic syndrome, insulin resistance, prediabetes, hyperinsulinemia, and fatty liver (NAFLD). Left to progress, I faced a future of type 2 diabetes, heart disease, high blood pressure, dialysis, and neuropathy, to name a few. Not to mention, I stared down an early grave before I even reached my fiftieth birthday.

In addition to those major issues, don't forget my other ailments: migraines and daily headaches, cystic acne, skin-picking (related to trichotillomania), acid reflux, joint inflammation and pain, painful periods, ovarian cysts, insomnia, foul mood, exercise-induced asthma, frequent colds, coughs, and cases of flu.

Emotionally, I was battling wild mood swings and emotional, mindless eating. The professionals told me to eat five to six times daily, which mentally permitted me to eat at any time of the day, even when I was not hungry. I'll share much more about the emotional battles in the next section, but I wanted to weave the mindless eating in with my physical symptoms because I had no idea how to recognize true hunger. All I knew was that I was craving carbohydrates all day, hungry or not. Spiritually, I had absolutely no idea I was craving so much more in my soul. There will be much more about our spiritual health in the final section, "Redeeming Your Spirit."

I know it seems like a lot of challenging diagnoses. And you may battle many more than the ones I mentioned. Perhaps you have already been diagnosed with type 2 diabetes. But it's not too late to change your course. Don't give up hope now, dear friend!

The remarkable story, full of God-incidences, of my battle against this metabolic mess follows. I may have been struck down and out for three decades, but what lies ahead in my journey is full of miracles, turnarounds, and victories! In sharing my life-changing weight-loss method with friends and families (and coaching clients through *The SugarFreed Me Weight-Loss Solution* program)—I am positive you will find victories in your journey.

Let's explore how you, too, can find hope for healing—physically, emotionally, and spiritually—body, mind, heart, and soul.

Coincidently, I learned about my NAFLD diagnosis right around the same time I started using my CPAP machine. Because of my improved sleep, I had more energy each day. If you are overweight and exhausted, please call for a sleep study. Perhaps that will be your transform-action task for this chapter.

Now that we've confronted the hard truths about our health, we must take our next step. Let's go!

A Note to Your Former Self:

A Note to Your Future Self:

Transform-Action Task:

CHAPTER 5

LEARNING A NEW LIFESTYLE: LIVING SUGAR*FREED*

■ ■ ■

You've set your resolve and confronted your own chronic health issues. Now it's time for you to learn the practical steps to live the Sugar*Freed* lifestyle. Remember my saying, *learn the science, apply the science, and change your life*? It's time to act.

In addition to advocating fasting for health, Dr. Fung suggests following a low-carb eating method to unlock the secrets to your obesity and finally find freedom and victory in your weight-loss battle. This advice is especially for those with severe insulin resistance (me), type 2 diabetes (almost me), prediabetes (me), metabolic syndrome (me), hyperinsulinemia (me), and just plain old belly fat accumulation (me, me, me)! My friend, if you have belly fat, you most likely have some level of insulin resistance, which impedes your weight-loss goals.

I desired quick healing, so I immediately jumped into this Sugar*Freed*, low-carb lifestyle suggestion. And because I had a lot of weight to lose, I chose an aggressive approach with my choice of daily carbohydrates. My new way of eating limited carbohydrates to twenty grams or less daily. Yes, it represented a drastic switch, but I found the transition easier because I had already quit white sugar and refined carbohydrates (processed factory foods).

After my late night of bingeing on Dr. Fung's videos, I subscribed to my new favorite website, *DietDoctor.com*, and signed up for a two-week challenge to get started. I picked a handful of the recipes in the challenge and dedicated myself to their plan for those first two weeks. I tweaked it based on something new I learned that evening. Dr. Fung mentioned that you should only eat when you are hungry. I've never felt hungry in the morning, so from then on, I chose to stop eating breakfast, contrary to the instructions given by other diet plans I had followed for years.

For fun, I entered my typical so-called *healthy* breakfast into my tracking app, *CarbManager*. Before my Sugar*Freed* lifestyle, I would start each day with a half cup of steel-cut oats, a half cup of fresh blueberries, and a drizzle of brown rice syrup. *Unbelievable!* Every morning, I ate more carbohydrates (carbs) than I do now in four days. Completely mind-blowing and somewhat depressing. Below is the macronutrient breakdown of this daily oatmeal breakfast.

Steel-cut oatmeal (1/2 cup), Blueberries (1/2 cup), and Brown Rice Syrup (1 tablespoon):

Protein: 9 grams

Fat: 4 grams

Carbohydrates: 73 grams

I have absolutely no doubt in my mind that my blood sugar would skyrocket every morning. Here's the real crazy part: *I wasn't even hungry.* However, I was following the diet plan of a diabetes prevention program. How in the world would a breakfast like this prevent type 2 diabetes? This breakfast was part of a recommended diet to *eat five to six meals daily to keep the metabolism active.* I'm positive you are familiar with this dietary advice.

I never thought to ask, "What if I'm not hungry?" I was captive to the dietary dogma that failed my metabolic health for decades. Are you ready to ditch the standard dietary dogma to break free in your weight-loss endeavor?

One five-minute video completely changed my life. I no longer wanted to be a sugar burner for fuel. Dr. Fung instructed me to turn my body into a fat-burning machine. It's all because of a random Google search. I praise God for prompting me to follow up on my earlier conversation with my friend that Friday evening. After a long week of work, I was exhausted but ended up reading and watching content from Dr. Fung into the wee hours of the night. I've never had a hero before, but I call Dr. Fung my earthly *health hero*. God is transforming lives through Dr. Fung's work.

The idea of fasting was not completely foreign to me. I knew the story of Jesus fasting for forty days and nights and then being tempted by Satan in the book of Luke.

> Jesus, full of the Holy Spirit, returned from the Jordan and was led by the Spirit into the desert, where for forty days he was tempted by the devil. He ate nothing during those days, and at the end of them he was hungry. The devil said to him, "If you are the Son of God, tell this stone to become bread." Jesus answered, "It is written: 'Man shall not live on bread alone.'" (Luke 4:1–4)

I have friends who have completed fasts for spiritual reasons, but I never imagined being capable of completing a fast. I was certain I would starve, so I always recused myself from participating. But fasting as a fat burner? Intriguing! I readily trusted Jesus's reminder: *I do not live on bread alone.*

With my new knowledge about my insulin hormone, I began to apply the life-changing science of fasting and low-carb food to my daily nourishment. The result of my two-week challenge? A ten-pound weight loss! Crazy, I know. Crazy and exciting. It confirmed the truth when Dr. Fung said, "This is not your fault." But taking on the responsibility, I quickly confirmed the low-carb way of eating is exactly what my metabolically deranged body needed.

See what I did there? I *learned* the science. I immediately *applied* the science. And I quickly *changed* my life. Remember this: *Learn. Apply. Change.* This is like no other way of eating you have ever tried before. I've had a few results in dieting with some weight loss, but I never found anything that made me feel the way I feel following a Sugar*Freed* lifestyle. Feelings of boundless energy and extreme productivity. Feelings of empowerment and a new ability to control hunger and *cravings*. Feeling free from the *sugar shackles* for the first time in my life! Let me explain how this worked, beginning with the physiological reactions to ditching sugar and carbs.

Remember the rollercoaster ride of our blood sugar? Up and down all day long as we feed our body five to six times daily with SAD. I immediately stopped that wild ride by drastically cutting my carbohydrate intake. I went from eating a daily breakfast of almost eighty grams of carbohydrates to less than twenty grams of carbohydrates daily. Drastic? Yes. Impossible? Absolutely not! If I did it, you can do it.

I devoured blog posts by good doctors like Dr. Fung. I streamed You-Tube videos when I couldn't read. I followed podcasts. I did not keep track, but I have invested hundreds of hours in learning the science to change my life. And now I know I've invested those hours to support you. For a list of recommended resources, visit the Resources page for a QR code you can scan on your phone or tablet.

As a side note, I wish I had discovered my functional medicine doctor before I embarked on this journey, but I'm delighted to have found her shortly afterward. I strongly recommend that you find a *low-carb-friendly* doctor. I felt a little alone in my journey to start, and there's a lot to be said for a great support system—beginning with a great, supportive doctor. And a passionate *Certified Christian Health and Wellness Coach* for education and accountability—me!

Thankfully, my cardiologist sparked the idea of low-carb living in my head. After I told him I was on a journey to "quit sugar," he replied, "Great, now quit bread, pasta, and potatoes, too, and watch your health change!" That's right—my cardiologist recommended low-carb living for me before I even knew it was a thing. I thought he was crazy at the time because standard dietary advice includes whole-grain bread, pasta, and potatoes. Right? What interesting advice he provided during that visit. Unfortunately, it would be several months before I watched Dr. Fung and truly understood what my cardiologist meant. But eventually, I did arrive at quitting bread, pasta, and potatoes. What happened when I arrived?

The severe leveling out of my blood sugars and insulin immediately improved my health, with obvious weight loss on the scale. But most importantly, for someone starting on another *crazy* (crazy good!) diet, I quickly realized that I had tamed my wild cravings for sugary and savory carbohydrates like chips and chocolate! I began to recognize the fact that I was *not* hungry all the time. I'm never *hangry* (you know, hungry + angry = *hangry*) following this way of eating. It's a crazy but true-blue miracle.

I hear people lament that such a drastic cut in carbohydrate consumption would never work for them. I like to encourage them with my truth about the physiological results of eliminating excessive sugar (carbs) from my daily life. First, I committed to trying it for two weeks through my challenge. If I can commit to two weeks, I encourage anyone else to try it for two weeks. I'm here to support everyone in this effort to ensure you don't feel alone in your journey.

Speaking of people lamenting, I'm excited to introduce you to the first of six stories from my coaching clients. I'll never forget the first conversation Deborah and I had regarding her health.

"I don't know, Christine. I'm from the South and don't know if I could ever give up my sweet tea!" Deborah lamented.

I smirked because I knew she would eventually have to face this fact. As I sensed her resolve to regain control of her health, I suspected that sweet tea would be the story of her past. I instantly knew this would be her "ditching coffee cold turkey" moment, her line in the sand, her first choice.

Deborah was living daily with autoimmune pain and walking with a cane. God had impressed on her heart that living in constant pain wasn't normal or healthy. And although she didn't have a lot of weight to lose, she decided that quitting sugar might alleviate some of that pain. So, after our conversation, Deborah dove in feet first into a twenty-one-day challenge to bust her sugar cravings. I'll let her share her story in her own words.

———

Deborah Malone's Story—Reduce the Pain, Ditch the Cane!
When I decided to connect with Coach Christine, I was facing total knee replacement surgery. Three months out from surgery, I was using a cane and feeling very old. I knew something needed to change, so I jumped on Coach Christine's train to healthy living.

Over a few months, I had so many positive changes in my life. My pain level went down. I no longer need a cane. I started walking in nature, and

I lost fifteen pounds that I didn't even know I needed to lose! I'm almost seventy years old and here to tell you that change does not depend on age.

Was it easy? Not really, but Coach Christine's passionate help and her community encouraged me to succeed. The women in this faith-based community get what I'm going through and long for the same results!

I am so thankful I decided to stick with her plan to bust my sugar cravings and experience so many positive changes in my life. As I move into my winter season, I have more energy and joy to step up and step out confidently into the calling God has placed on my life as an author and speaker.

———

How amazing! Deborah ditched her sweet tea for good in just a few days and now drinks infused water.

And what's more impressive is that she went from relying on her cane to ditching it! I trust that Deborah's story will provide hope that living pain-free, losing weight, and busting your sugar cravings are doable.

This all began when Deborah made her first choice. And she quickly learned that yes, *yes*, she could live without her sweet tea. That tiny choice delivered significant results for her.

Deborah made it happen.

The result of our commitment to our health?

Deborah and I have been set *free*! SugarFreed, to be exact. We are free from up-and-down blood sugar rollercoaster swings, reducing our pain, and getting in touch with the actual signs of physical hunger. Controlling cravings *and* realizing we don't have to eat all day long. And we can live without coffee and sweet tea loaded with sugar!

Yes, it's true. Pinch me, please. Almost thirty years of chronic dieting and constantly feeling hungry and moody left me skeptical that I would ever heal my body. I forgot to mention that Deborah was skeptical, too. I heard it in her tone when she said, "Well, I don't know, Christine," but Deborah and I were total believers after two short weeks of committing to living SugarFreed through a low-carb way of eating.

Now, how about you? What can you look forward to as you dive in and learn to love this new lifestyle?

Your insulin hormone health will improve if you reduce your blood sugars daily (by eliminating high-carb intake). Your body will cease screaming at you to be fed around the clock. This embodies the basic science of low-carb living. I like to say, "It's all about the hormones, baby!"

I hear you lamenting in your mind—does that mean I have to give up some of my staple foods? Yeah, yeah—most likely, if those foods are high in sugar or carbohydrates—you'll need to ditch them.

However, as an eternal optimist, I remind you to focus on what you *can* eat. Because I swear to you, once you control your cravings and hunger, you will drastically reduce your *physical* cravings for foods high in sugar. Those foods keep us fat. Remember, insulin is our fat-storing hormone.

What we *can* eat is wholesome food from *God's good smorgasbord*! You can find this food on the perimeter of the grocery store. You can purchase food from your local farmer. You can even raise it or grow it yourself! If you're raising your grass-fed beef, pork, or chicken, let me say you are so blessed! This reminds me of another favorite psalm to enjoy during your Sugar*Freed* journey:

> Because your love is better than life,
> my lips will glorify you.
> I will praise you as long as I live,
> and in your name I will lift up my hands.
> My soul will be satisfied as with the
> richest of foods;
> with singing lips my mouth will praise you.
> —Psalm 63:3–5

As a follower of healthy fats and a low-carb diet, can you see how our hearts will sing? We get to enjoy the *richest, the fattiest of foods*, like beef, pork, fatty fish, and bacon. All the natural, whole foods created by our Creator. How incredibly satisfying is God's good smorgasbord!

Thinking about how much I now enjoy the entire process of nourishing my body causes me to pause as I recall my former trips to the grocery store. I despised grocery shopping while feeding myself and my family the SAD diet. Hundreds of dollars spent on boxed and factory-processed foods used to annoy me. At the time, I was into the convenience of it all. A victim of food-and-diet marketing scams, I spent far too much money on *Weight Watchers* frozen desserts and Lean Cuisine meals. Did any of those packaged items leave me full and satisfied? No. They skyrocketed my blood sugar with their high-carb content and then crashed my blood sugar two hours later. Those *convenient meals* always left me wondering where my next meal would come from. They left me craving more, enslaved, and offered me an excuse to keep up the *five-to-six meals daily routine,* which continued to wreak havoc on my carbohydrate-intolerant metabolism.

Now when I grocery shop, I find joy in the process. I whiz through the store in record time because one of the key strategies and benefits of low-carb living is that you only mostly shop the perimeter of the store. That's right, you don't have to spend an hour going up and down each store aisle. The edge of the store stocks all you need: fresh produce, meat and deli counters, cheese, dairy, and eggs. Look how much time we save! I rarely venture into the middle aisles anymore. The only reason to venture into the center of the store is for items like coffee, tea, spices, sugar-free condiments, pickles, and olives.

There are two fundamental practices I follow for eating a low-carb lifestyle:

1. Always read *ingredient* labels (look for any sugar and seed oils—avoid them).
2. Check the nutritional information on carbohydrates per serving.

These are some food ideas to satisfy your physical hunger (this list is not all-inclusive):

> **Dairy and Eggs:** butter, heavy cream, heavy whipping cream, cream cheese, mascarpone cheese, hard cheeses, sour cream, ricotta cheese, plain Greek yogurt, eggs
> **Meat and Deli:** bacon, ground beef, beef chuck roasts, beef steaks (ribeye, strip, filet mignon), poultry, pork shoulder or butt, pork tenderloin, pork chops, sausage, lunch meat (check sausage and deli item ingredients carefully to avoid added sugar)

Fish/Seafood: salmon, shrimp, lobster, crab legs, scallops, fish, tuna, sardines

Vegetables: *Often*–cauliflower, broccoli, brussels sprouts, asparagus, leafy greens

Occasionally–green, red, yellow, orange bell peppers, onion

Fruits: *Often*–avocado

Occasionally—blackberries, raspberries, strawberries, tomatoes

Nuts: *Occasionally*—pecans, walnuts, almonds, macadamia

Condiments: mustard, avocado mayonnaise, sugar-free dressing and sauces, apple cider vinegar, spices, and seasonings (check item ingredients to avoid added sugar)

Oils: avocado oil, olive oil, coconut oil, bacon grease, beef tallow, ghee

Low-carb replacement items: *Occasionally*—almond flour, coconut flour, and Sukrin USA sugar substitute products (you can find a link to my favorite low-carb pantry items in my Amazon shop included in my resources for you.)

Packaged foods: pickles, olives, bone broth, canned tomato products like salsa, marinara sauce, diced, and paste (*essential* to check ingredients—watch for sneaky sugars)

Beverages: water, coffee, sparkling water, occasional spirits, and dry red or white wine (search for clean-crafted wine with no added sugar, dyes, or chemicals)

(For a downloadable copy of my grocery shopping list, scan the QR code on the Resources page.)

Do you find it crazy that all my food choices fit on one page? Something I've learned on this journey, and I enjoy implementing, is this: *keep it super simple.* You know the acronym *KISS?* This list of foods is my go-to. It keeps me super satiated and super satisfied while being super simple. I whiz in and out of the grocery store in no time now. Hooray! Believe it or not, our grocery bills each month are also lower. I spend more for quality, nutrient-rich food but save money because the overall quantity of food is much less. Quality over quantity!

Here's another valid point I share with new low-carb people. As you look over my list above, you may think, "Wow, that's not a lot of options," but trust me on this. Eventually, your mindset will transform to realize a secret and easy formula: *Food is fuel.* It's truly a simple formula I realized after I flipped my cravings and learned to recognize true hunger to satisfy my *physical* needs. You bet there's a huge *emotional* and *spiritual* process to journey through, which we will cover, but remember: **This is a journey of the heart, the wellspring of our life.**

When it comes to healing your metabolism physically, I firmly believe that a diet high in sugar and carbohydrates *triggers cravings* for the wrong foods throughout the day. Even if marketed as a *WeightWatchers* treat, the food won't effectively satisfy your cravings or hunger. It will only launch you on that wild rollercoaster ride of overconsumption, blood sugar swings, and crazy food cravings. I no longer need that thrill in my life. I got off that ride! Want to join me?

How can I persuade you to try this low-carb lifestyle for your healing? The Sugar*Freed* lifestyle combined with intermittent fasting healed my body. I bet my stories of healing will be your story too. Let's explore more how to make this big ditch and switch in the next chapter.

A Note to Your Former Self:

A Note to Your Future Self:

Transform-Action Task:

CHAPTER 6

DITCHING SUGAR:

SWITCHING TO FAT FOR FUEL

Ready to receive your marching orders? I won't sugarcoat this (see what I did there?). This battle will be one of the toughest challenges of your life. Most likely, you have dedicated yourself to losing weight and found some success with traditional diets. Today, I need you to ditch the word *diet* from your vocabulary. We are launching into a *lifestyle*—one that will stick and give you lasting victory. To win, we need a solid battle plan. Planning and goal-setting come naturally for this Type-A author, so I'm privileged to add these steps to your journey.

The lifestyle lessons that stick, the daily drills, if you will, will deliver lifetime results. These daily routines are the keys to our success.

"Christine, how in the world can you maintain your health and weight-loss success day after day?" Women ask me this question all the time because we are prone to wander and fail repeatedly. I can vividly recall the days of yo-yo dieting, but no more.

I consistently practice *five hard and fast rules for success*. These rules have ushered in my weight-loss victory and allowed me to maintain weight loss without questioning my future health. I am also humbled and honored to write these drill instructions for your victory.

Hard. Yes, I said hard. Remember, weight-loss success is a matter of the heart. Our hearts can be so hard—including my own. Don't think I'm singling you out. Interestingly enough, I have studied the book of Ezekiel twice through my health journey, and this verse I share is a reminder of what God has in store for you. Write it down and hold it close in your heart.

> I will give you a new heart and put a new spirit in you; I will remove from you your heart of stone and give you a heart of flesh. And I will put my Spirit in you and move you to follow my decrees and be careful to keep my laws. (Ezekiel 36:26–27)

You are about to embark on a way of caring for your health that incorporates your body, mind, and spirit. We will discuss mind and spirit in the following two sections, but allow me to share these five practical rules that will impact your weight-loss journey. I call these my *Five Lifestyle Rules for Success*. They worked for me; they will serve you well, too.

Lifestyle Rule #1: Learn the Science, Apply the Science, and Change Your Life

I opened this book with my mantra: *learn the science, apply the science, and change your life*. This concept offers an integral part of your journey—*the buy-in*! Your willingness to learn a new approach to food and sugar and how the wrong types of food impact your blood sugar, hormones, and overall health will change your life. But you do have to act (recall that *action* is a part of the heart transformation). That's where the *application of science* comes into play. In this lifestyle lesson, I want to share my most crucial science practices and some of my favorite resources.

I don't want to overwhelm you with all the resources I have used over the years (I have invested hundreds of hours geeking out on the science of a low-carb, Sugar*Freed* lifestyle), so I will share the first five resources that put me on this path to freedom. For more of my most trusted resources, please scan the QR code on the Resources page.

My Top Five SugarFreed Resources

1. *DietDoctor.com*. This is my number-one go-to website and is the world's largest low-carb website available today. This site offers a

well-rounded variety of experts in the field. This site does not just provide a one-size-fits-all approach to this lifestyle. I appreciate the voices on this platform who may not all agree expressly on a topic, such as protein intake. During my weight-loss months, I followed the advice for a strict keto way of eating and kept to a daily protein ratio of 25 percent (and 5 percent carbohydrates and 70 percent healthy fats). This ratio worked for me to achieve a healthy weight. However, as menopause kicked in, I dialed back on the fat intake and upped my protein intake for my aging body and metabolism. My ratios are now 30 to 35 percent protein, 5 percent carbs, and 60 to 65 percent healthy fats.

DietDoctor.com supports both approaches through the various experts featured, including videos, blog posts, great recipes, personal challenges, and more. I am always delighted to remind Dr. Andreas Eenfeldt (the founder of the site) of just how much good he has done worldwide. His vision will help you too. I fully endorse the annual membership, as well. It's inexpensive, plus the science resources are endless.

2. *The Obesity Code: Unlocking the Secrets of Weight Loss* by Jason Fung, MD, is the book (besides my Bible) that changed my health. If you are not a reader, I urge you to listen to it in audiobook. Dr. Fung's book provides hope (as I described in the intro chapters—remember, this is not entirely your fault!) and a carefully written science-based and science-backed guide to unlocking the secrets of your obesity. And he wrote it for a non-scientist to understand easily. Dr. Fung and Dr. Eenfeldt are my earthly health heroes. I will never be able to repay them for the knowledge they instilled in my life. How can you put a price on *freedom*?

3. *Why We Get Fat and What to Do About It* by Gary Taubes. I highly recommend reading this book after *The Obesity Code*. Gary is an investigative journalist with an interest in science and health. This book is a national bestseller and answers the question from the book's title. It revealed the dysfunction in our dietary guidelines and how Western societies market mass-produced, hyper-palatable junk as food. After reading these two books, I quickly and easily

dumped the old dietary dogma of *calories in, calories out; eating less and moving more;* and *everything in moderation.*

4. *Ken D. Berry, MD, YouTube Channel.* Dr. Berry is one of my favorite doctors to watch on YouTube (author of *Lies My Doctor Told Me*). His videos are short, educational, and filled with some cheeky humor with quips like "That's just dumb…" regarding old dietary advice that is keeping you sick! YouTube is an excellent resource for learning lessons about the Sugar*Freed* lifestyle. I invite you to subscribe to my YouTube channel under my name, where I share real-life tips and inspiration along with testimonial interviews with my clients. (youtube.com/christinetrimpe)

5. *X (formerly Twitter) Low-Carb Community.* My final recommendation on this short list of resources is X, where you will find a very supportive and engaging low-carb community. Follow me and check out the people I regularly engage with or retweet, like Brian Lenzkes, MD (host of "Life's Best Medicine Podcast") and Cynthia Thurlow, NP (host of "Everyday Wellness Podcast"). Cynthia is the author of the bestseller *Intermittent Fasting Transformation.* Cynthia specializes in fasting for women and hormonal health. Be sure to follow Cynthia and Dr. Lenzkes.

The resources are there for you. Will you commit to learning? But don't get stuck in the learning, learning, learning phase. That leads to procrastination. Learn something today (from this book) and commit to applying it now. This brings us to my next rule for success. Take what you've learned and set your goals.

Lifestyle Rule #2: Always Have a Plan

Remember, we are on a path to victory, running a marathon. It's not a sprint. But you need to have a purpose and a plan for what victory looks like. Most importantly, remember this is a journey for life, so while the ultimate *outcome* is a great goal, I prefer to coach you through your daily *output.*

We must fix our gaze and focus forward. Add blinders to help you stay the course, and for heaven's sake, know that you can learn from the past, *but it's time to stop living in the past.* That plan didn't work out so well for either of us, did it?

It is now time for you to step into the plans that God has for your health. Write out this verse and put it in front of your face every day.

> Therefore, since we are surrounded by such a great cloud of witnesses, let us throw off everything that hinders and the sin that so easily entangles, and let us run with perseverance the race marked out for us. Let us fix our eyes on Jesus, the author and perfecter of our faith, who for the joy set before him endured the cross, scorning its shame, and sat down at the right hand of the throne of God. (Hebrews 12:1–2)

That's an excellent plan to follow and is confirmed repeatedly in my coaching. This passage of Scripture provides encouragement (the great cloud of witnesses), direction (throw off hindrances), structure (run with perseverance), and how to stay focused on your goals (eyes fixed on Jesus). Jesus completed the hardest task known to mankind with a heart of joy for you. Don't miss that He has scorned the shame of the horrific trial He endured, and His work is complete on your behalf. What joy it is to understand that God does have a plan for your life! Now, how will you respond?

Join God where He is working around you and watch Him work out His plan for your life and the healthy new you in ways you least expect. Lean on the Lord daily for guidance in your personal health goals. God will direct you in your plans. He even cares about your life's simple, mundane parts, like meal planning, fitness routines, and tracking your progress.

Let's make a pact—you and me. You will invite the Lord into your planning stages and then act and go where He leads. Letting God guide you will bring about His glory in your success. "So whether you eat or drink or whatever you do, do it all for the glory of God" (1 Corinthians 10:31).

Speaking of making a pact, goal-setting involves a mindset shift or focus on how you approach your weight-loss goals. I coach my preferred goal-setting strategies through the PACT method. In chapter 7, "Marching Forward in Victory," I will explain this PACT strategy in more detail.

In the meantime, start outlining your plan and asking yourself what words like discipline, determination, and perseverance will mean to your desired outcome.

Lifestyle Rule #3: Practice Time-Restricted Eating—Stop Eating Around the Clock!

Per Dr. Fung, the number one rule of the time-restricted *eating club* (also known as fasting or intermittent fasting) is to not talk about the club! But I must. It could be the best tool to set you free in your physical, emotional, and spiritual health. In this book, I will encourage you to begin adopting a *time-restricted eating* (TRE) lifestyle and to commence this practice today.

TRE will free you from the old dietary advice to eat all day to keep your metabolism revving. Trust me when I tell you this is terrible advice for those of us who struggle with obesity due to insulin resistance.

Ask yourself, "Why am I eating when I'm not hungry?" My TRE journey began as soon as I watched a few Dr. Fung videos, and he said, "That's just dumb," regarding eating when not hungry. I did not eat breakfast the following day because I was not hungry. I had my break-*fast* around 11:30 a.m. and fell into a natural eating pattern only when I was hungry—11:30 a.m. and 5:30 p.m. This was my initial success with TRE. Avoiding food when I was not hungry gave me the first taste of this food freedom journey.

As a result of the fantastic benefits of TRE, one of my primary coaching philosophies is "*Stop eating around the clock!*" Eating satiating SugarFreed meals only when I was hungry brought on weight loss, and I testify it also ushered in the incredible gift of self-control. Self-control—that fruit of the spirit we'd rather not pursue or even draw attention to in our lives. Our society accepts eating around the clock. They promote it! It's part of the standard dietary advice, for crying out loud. And it caused frustration and kept me fat for decades.

Physically, my blood sugar and insulin hormone were out of control, contributing to my morbid obesity.

Emotionally, it permitted me to eat my feelings. "Oh hey, I'm supposed to eat all day to keep this *mysterious metabolism* running. Right?"

Spiritually, I easily overlooked the acceptable sin of gluttony. I did not understand how God guides and calls us to treat our temple. When the lightbulb illuminated how I approached meal timing for my body, mind, and spirit, I was in for a substantial, life-changing lesson. In the next section, let's explore the topic of overeating, overindulging, and gluttony at a deeper level.

If you're anything like me, you've heard of people fasting, but you can't fathom going without food for any length of time. Hey, I know. I thought those fasting people were a little kooky, but again, I did not understand the depth of the power of fasting first for our spiritual health while also providing excellent benefits for our physical health. Next, I will share how to face periods of fasting without spiraling into episodes of *hangry*.

Lifestyle Rule #4: Choose Foods That Satiate and Satisfy

This rule is of utmost importance. It will prevent you from living the *hangry* life you've lived all these years in your dieting endeavors. I don't know about you, but I despise being *hangry*. Based on my mood while *hangry*, I'm sure my family hates it too!

I have found freedom from getting *hangry* by learning to choose foods that truly satiate and satisfy my hunger—and I'm referring to the hunger of my body, mind, and spirit. I had been craving all the wrong things to satisfy my soul.

The day I discovered *DietDoctor.com*, I found the people on that website eating bacon. What?!? They were talking about filling up on bacon. How bizarre. Haven't we been warned (and shamed) about eating bacon? Bacon is supposed to make us fat. However, I am pleased to share that I lost one hundred pounds while eating bacon. And I ate a lot of bacon during my weight-loss journey. I could go on and on about bacon. Bacon is the symbol to me of the ultimate ditch-and-switch success. I ditched the dietary dogma that bacon makes me fat and opened my mind to a new approach—choose foods that satiate and satisfy.

I've already shared in depth what this means regarding what to throw in your grocery cart, but I just wanted to highlight this and tell you that you can avoid living *hangry*. Remember those calorie restriction days?

Remember those *Weight Watchers* frozen desserts that left you wanting more? Those choices never satiate and satisfy! Now is the time to open your mind to nutrient-rich foods, full of healthy fats and not loaded with sugar.

Imagine my delight to read about satiating and satisfying food from God's good smorgasbord throughout Scripture. Check this out. Can you smell the aroma of the cooking fat? "My soul will be satisfied as with the richest of foods; with singing lips my mouth will praise you" (Psalm 63:5). David is writing about marrow and fat!

Healthy fats and protein satiate and satisfy and are critical to ditching sugar. They are instrumental to your success and will help you gain control over what goes in your mouth. This leads me to my last hard-and-fast lifestyle rule.

Lifestyle Rule #5: Live Within Your Boundaries

Let me ask you a question. You probably know the answer, but I ask it every day: "Is it easier to *stay on track* or *get back on track?*"

If you picked *stay on track*, ding-ding-ding! You know the correct answer. Yes, why, oh, why do we continually self-sabotage?

The answer lies somewhere between the characteristics of the heart transformation I explained in with the HEART acronym in chapter 2. Let's review those characteristics and see if you can spot where you need some support.

What's a typical result when we fail to *handle our emotions*? We have breakdowns and hissy-fits and find a plethora of excuses to comfort ourselves with food.

And then, we berate ourselves for our moment of weakness and fail to *examine how damaging these invasive thoughts* are to our well-being.

Then, we give up again and fail to see how we lack *motivation* to care for our health in a way that glorifies God.

Guilt and shame pile up, and we aren't *running with courage*. We are hiding out, hoping no one will notice how far off the tracks we have plummeted.

Paralyzed once again, we are in no place to *act*.

My friend, do not despair. I understand exactly how you feel. However, I can tell you that you can overcome this cycle of repeatedly falling off track when you accept and embrace the concept of boundaries. Now, I could probably write an entire book on living within the boundary lines of pleasant places with the Lord—but for brevity's sake, let me explain what I mean regarding your weight-loss goals with an example from my life.

A significant component of my coaching philosophy requires clients to regularly set new boundaries as they progress in their weight-loss journey. I have complete confidence in this coaching technique because of my experience with making choices. As I set out to quit sugar, I spaced out my choices, my new boundary line, every few days. Soon, I realized that I was successfully living the Sugar*Freed* lifestyle. I busted my sugar cravings within a few short weeks!

Let's call these boundary lines small habit changes, which changed my approach to gaining victory in my weight-loss goals. *Small habit changes build and deliver big results.* You can quote me on that! I experienced it in my journey, and I see it play out daily in the clients I coach.

The ultimate goal of the Sugar*Freed* way of living is enjoying the fact that we no longer crave sugar. Living within your boundaries requires that you know your limits. You don't want to bust your boundaries and fall off track again.

In December 2019, I had lived at my weight-loss goal for almost two years. As my daughter's December wedding approached, people began to ask me if I would eat a piece the wedding cake. Now, up until that point, I had abstained from desserts that contained sugar. But you know what? I paid $600 for that cake, so I was wondering what made that cake so special. Would I eat a piece of this cake? That was the question only I could answer for myself.

Would I cross my boundary line of living a 100 percent Sugar*Freed* lifestyle? If I did decide to eat the cake, would it throw me completely off track? Did I want to take the risk? What if eating the cake would require months to get back on track?

These are all important questions you will also ask yourself as you go through your weight-loss journey. You will need to consider your track record. I considered my track record of the many failed attempts in my weight-loss struggles.

But this time, my friend, something was very different in my weight-loss journey. This time, due to another one of my hard-and-fast lifestyle rules, *eating satiating and satisfying foods*, I knew that I could fall back on the lifestyle choices I had made during my Sugar*Freed* journey.

I was 100 percent confident that if I did eat a piece of wedding cake, I would not fall off track and back into a sugar or food binge. So, I ate a piece of the cake. And guess what? It was super sweet (your tastebuds will change, believe me). I also ended up bringing home a full sheet of extra cake. Did I eat that? No. I sent it home with the wedding guests.

I had consciously decided to eat one piece of wedding cake, and I didn't even finish it because I was enjoying my time with friends and family (not food). I stuck by my choice to eat only one piece. Living within my boundaries for a long time made this easier, setting me up for success in that decision.

This illustrates the importance of having firm boundaries in place with your goal to gain victory in your weight-loss battle. I often remind my children that God gives us boundaries for a reason: to protect our hearts, which are so easily broken! Are you ready to progress in this heart transformation journey and live within your boundaries? Take heart with this promise from one of my favorites, a joy-filled psalm:

> LORD, you have assigned me my portion and my cup;
> you have made my lot secure.
> The boundary lines have fallen for me in pleasant places;
> surely I have a delightful inheritance.
> I will praise the LORD, who counsels me; even
> at night my heart instructs me.
> I have set the LORD always before me. Because he is at my right hand,
> I will not be shaken.
> —Psalm 16:5–8

These five lifestyle rules resulted in the victory over my obesity and chronic diseases that kept me in bondage for three decades. You can't unsee this newfound freedom once you *see, taste,* and *feel* these results. These practices will usher in a path to freedom, to finally taste and see what the

Lord has for you in your health and wellness—a healthy body, a clear mind, and a heart of passion in your spiritual journey with Jesus. These practices are achievable, attainable, and available when you choose to ditch sugar and refined carbohydrates from your way of eating. I call it the great ditch-and-switch because living Sugar*Freed* is great. You will feel better physically, emotionally, and spiritually as you lean on God for His guidance over your health. And by ditching a diet high in carbohydrates, you will turn into a fat-burning machine. Isn't that some great fuel for your fire?

Let's review my top five Sugar*Freed* rules:

1. Learn the Science, Apply the Science, and Change Your Life
2. Always Have a Plan
3. Practice Time-Restricted Eating—Don't Eat Around the Clock!
4. Choose Foods that Satiate and Satisfy
5. Live Within Your Boundaries

Now that you've equipped yourself with helpful lifestyle rules that bring success and freedom take some time to develop a few more of your own rules for success.

Don't stop now—it's time to march forth, and I will give you more motivation in the next chapter.

A Note to Your Former Self:

A Note to Your Future Self:

Transform-Action Task:

CHAPTER 7

MARCHING FORWARD IN VICTORY

You are armed with the strategies and may think this sounds good, but you're weary of marching in this weight-loss battle. I know. But I promise, the marching takes on a rhythm that moves you toward victory (significantly as you drop the excess weight of fat, guilt, and shame).

Motivation is critical to winning this battle. And don't forget motivation is a vital component of a heart transformation. Since motivation is a word we understand but struggle to define, I'll share the definition again and remind you of this step in our HEART acronym: *Ask for Motivation.*

The definition of motivation is a motivating force, stimulus, or influence.[22] "What exactly would be a force, stimulus, and influence to inspire action?" Great question! In my journey and while observing my coaching clients, it's easy to see that you and I are motivated by many motivational techniques. And they work when you act. Now, let's build a list so you can check off motivational strategies that will work for you.

But first, let's arm ourselves with a battle cry as a banner over our mission. This verse strongly reminds us that the God of creation created our bodies for a purpose! "Do you not know that your body is a temple of the Holy Spirit, who is in you, whom you have received from God? You are not your own; you were bought at a price. Therefore honor God with your body" (1 Corinthians 6:19–20).

So then, what shall we do? Let's begin by asking God for the motivation to act, to see this journey through. To move, let's make a list from the definition of motivation.

An essential skill I have developed as a coach is determining the factors that motivate you to act (thus, motivation leads to the T in our heart transformation—Take Action). It will not surprise you that what motivates me may not motivate you. Motivation factors will be varied and can be external and internal. Let's explore by building a list specific to motivational forces, stimuli, and influence that will inspire you to act.

Motivational Forces

I didn't force you to pick up this book, but something sure did—perhaps the cover or the words on the back. Maybe you're familiar with my story. Perhaps you resonated with an inspiration I shared on social media. Maybe you read that I healed my fatty liver disease or defeated obesity and saw me on the cover of a magazine. Some force you may not even be able to put into words brought you to this page. I see five forces that played parts in my journey that may motivate you to act.

1. **Health Improvements.** Let's start with the obvious. We must pursue health improvements, simple as that. You've read about my progress and acknowledge that you must make progress, too. No doubt, losing weight will reduce the risk of chronic disease in the future, often reversing some of your diagnoses and, most importantly, improving your overall well-being. The fact that I no longer gasp for air when climbing stairs (or my beloved mountains) reminds me of my health improvements and that I must engage this motivational force daily.

2. **Quotes and Inspirational Messages**. Find a few favorites and plaster that inspiration everywhere! This force tends to work for everyone. While pursuing my goal weight, I still worked in a corporate office with a bunch of women. Treats and temptations filled our office space daily. I found this quote early in my journey and stuck it on my monitor. On my office door. In the breakroom and the lunchroom. And all over my home.
    "You can't go back and change the beginning,
    but you can start where you are and change the ending." —*Unknown*

I asked my Weight Loss by Faith community (see the resources for more information about my free Facebook Group) for their favorite inspirational quotes, and they came up with some excellent ones to share with you:

"Strive for progress, not perfection." —Unknown

"Your current situation is not your final destination." —Unknown

"Who you are tomorrow begins with what you do today." —Tim Fargo

"You are never too old to set another goal or to dream a new dream." —C. S. Lewis

"More things are wrought by prayer than this world dreams of." —Alfred Lord Tennyson

What inspiration will you write out and plaster everywhere? Ensure the theme motivates you to act, helps you progress in your goals, and gives you a vision of victory, leading you to the next force to engage in your journey.

3. **Vision of the Future.** This is the intent of a *Note to Your Future Self* at the end of each chapter. Ask yourself these questions. If I, Coach Christine, could wave a magic wand, and twelve months from now, you have overcome the struggles in your weight-loss journey, what does that look like to you? What are you now enjoying? How do you feel? What has changed? Describe what a perfect day looks like.

As the fog lifted early in my quitting-sugar journey, I began to have dreams of what a perfect day would look like for me at a healthy weight. My vision included simple things like bending over at the waist to tie my shoes without sitting down and having enough energy throughout the day so I didn't need to crawl into my bed when I got home from work. I pictured myself worshiping God on the mountain summits I would climb.

I also saw myself fitting in. Fitting in my cute clothes from the back of my closet to fitting in wherever and whenever I stepped out my front door to face the world. If I had to pick one word, it would be envisioning myself with a *new confidence*. My vision provided hope and a desire to be fully confident as a daughter of God, confident as I began to share this fantastic transformation, and confident in my new calling as an author, speaker, and coach.

What does that future perfect day look and feel like for you? How will you feel at your goal weight, and what does your life look like there?

4. **Positive Reinforcement.** It's no secret that we are women who like our rewards when we feel we've done something good or put in some extra hard work. I believe nothing is wrong with rewarding our positive movement toward our goals. Still, I've had to ditch my old reward system of a special food-related treat after counting calories or points all week. Nod your head in agreement with me here and answer me this: "Have you ever gone out for dessert with your *WeightWatchers* best friend after you've weighed in and sat through the meeting?" I'm guilty!

As you reach important milestones, might I suggest even more enticing rewards? How about a day at the spa? Or a pedicure? This was my favorite positive reinforcement reward. I was hitting up the thrift store for smaller clothes. I love the thrill of a bargain and buying clothes that now fit! And, of course, as you lose weight, you will need new clothes, so thrift shopping is the way to go. Here's a tip. Check out your local Salvation Army and search for brand-new clothing with tags. You will be surprised by what you can bring home.

Which one of these ideas reinforces a positive image in your mind? Do that!

5. **Success Stories**. When I discovered the *DietDoctor.com* website, I could spend hours on that site just reading the success stories. And no, that was not a waste of my time. Stories inspire everything about living this one life. We learn from stories, share stories, and listen when someone tells a great story. Stories have the power to change a life forever. Add a fantastic side-by-side transformation photo, and we can all agree that a picture is worth a thousand words of written story. Be sure to visit the Resources page for the link to a photo scrapbook of success stories.

My story is why I sat down to write to you. Stories still inspire me to pursue my health and wellness to the glory of God because who knows what part of a story will put someone else on a path to healing? I want to remind you why I've encouraged you to journal this journey. I pray your story will touch a life, too. Sara, my coaching client, shares her story below, and I'm honored to include it here for you now.

———

Sara Schaffer—My Story of SugarFreed Success

My doctor bluntly told me to lose twenty pounds. Frustrated, I asked, "How should I do that?" Her predictable answer, "Move more, eat less," pricked a familiar *been there, tried that* wound. My hope withered.

Six months later, Christine's social media posts caught my attention. I sensed a sincerity that intrigued me. As I researched, I found her program was biblically based. Curiosity piqued and hope returned, I enrolled in her Sugar*Freed Me* program.

I had *no idea* what I signed up for! The first few days weren't a diet regimen but prayer and Scripture meditation. Sitting with the Lord, I realized I was afraid to lose weight. Without exaggeration, I felt terrified. Old memories of painful words and abuse darkened my thoughts. If I were thin, I'd be vulnerable.

I prayed, and God showed me the truth: obesity couldn't keep me safe—He could. He gently asked to heal me. Medically, I was motivated to lose weight. Emotionally, I was ready to stop hiding. Spiritually, I was willing to believe and obey.

Soon after this, I discovered the definition of "sugar." In my cupboard, it included more than granulated white stuff. It also included popcorn. *Popcorn*!

For over eighteen years, my husband and I ate this *healthy snack* nightly, but then I learned it was the main thing I digested as I slept. My body was never getting the chance to burn fat. Would my husband feel hurt if I changed our routine?

Surprisingly, he quit popcorn when I told him I wouldn't eat anything after dinner. That was my first eating habit change, and I quickly lost weight.

Within a couple of months, I was swimming in my clothes. I went shopping and bravely grabbed a pair of jeans two sizes smaller than I was wearing. When I stepped out of the dressing room, an employee saw me and said, "Those are too big; you need a size smaller."

I stared at her. I heard the words but couldn't comprehend them. She handed me another pair. Incredulous, I returned to the dressing room and tried them on. They fit! After changing to my baggy clothes, I slung the three-sizes-smaller jeans over my arm. I walked around the store muttering, "I *am* this size," trying to believe what my eyes couldn't see.

Since then, I've lost over fifty pounds and celebrated what's true whether I feel it or not. When temptations come, I've learned to make coffee, keep decaf on hand for the afternoons, or distract myself with fifteen minutes of puzzles on my phone. Both are rewards to myself and shift my focus from food. Other favorite non-edible treats include napping, lighting candles, reading, and fresh flowers. The last three together are true luxury!

I've shed fifty pounds of fear. When it resurfaces, God reassures me. I no longer defend myself; I am hidden with Christ in God. He heals my past, handles my present, and holds my hope-filled future.

———

Thank you, Sara, for sharing your story! She forgot to mention that her husband also lost fifty pounds since Sara shared *The* Sugar*Freed Me Weight-Loss Solution* program with him. I call that a win-win: "Buy one, get one free!"

Motivational Stimuli

The amount of information our brain processes daily is mind-blowing (pun intended). Much of it we don't give a thought, but each day, we are bombarded with messages that may trigger or provoke us to take action to achieve our goals. When it comes to weight loss, this is very positive. We need the stimulus to move forward. Here are a few stimuli that I implemented for a positive outcome in my health.

1. **Goal Setting**. Super important! We can't arrive at a destination without a plan. In chapter six, I mentioned sharing my favorite goal-setting technique PACT, which stands for *Purposeful, Actionable, Continuous,* and *Trackable*. The philosophy behind this technique is *output-focused* rather than *outcome-focused*.

   What's the purpose of your weight-loss journey? Revisit your *why* questions and make a *purposeful* list. My current purpose in maintaining my weight loss is to keep my hormones balanced for sustainable weight loss, to reduce body fat percentage and build strength and muscle as I age (super important, ladies, to prevent falls and injury), and to eat a healthy diet for energy so I can show up daily for the calling that God has put on my life. I know that if I choose to eat a diet high in sugar and refined carbs, it will zap my energy. Just thinking about that exhausts me, so I am *purposeful* in my health goals for my body, mind, and spirit.

   You may lament right now, "But, Christine, it's hard. I don't know where to begin?" And we sit in that mindset and allow paralysis analysis to set in. Do you know what I'm talking about? It's that headspace where you know what to do, but could you? Will it work this time? Keep in mind that our hearts, our minds, our lives ... will not transform without that essential component of the heart transformation. *We must act.* It's time to form your *actionable* steps to get your desired results. So, write them down! Start today. It can be a considerable action or a start small action. But you must act. Am I right? I can coach and prod you until I'm blue in the face, but although I wish I could do the work for you (I've learned not to be afraid of the hard work), I simply can't. It's time for you to act.

   Here is a list of ideas for you: dedicate time to read this book and follow through on my suggestions, write down what you typically eat in a day, calculate the grams of sugar and carbs in your typical day, make a list of the food and drinks you consume that are high in sugar, decide what needs to go, block out your schedule this week to get in some minutes of movement, clean out your pantry and fridge of unhealthy food, plan your meals, start organizing your favorite healthy recipes, grocery shop the perimeter to prepare for the upcoming week, batch cook and freeze meals, check your blood sugar each morning or before and after meals, show up in my community for accountability, journal about your day and the impact on your health, book that doctor appointment you've been putting off, and … boy this list is getting long!

Basically, *do the thing*. Take action to transform your health. *Just do it* to borrow a common phrase. If you need more ideas, visit the Resources page for the link to grab my free guide: *Crush Your Cravings: The Ultimate Wellness Guide for Christian Women*. It contains tips you can implement today. Finally, write out your actionable steps if you haven't completed your *transform-action* tasks after each chapter.

2. **Progress Tracking**. "*You can't fix what you don't find.*" You can quote me on that. It's important to "find" where you are in your journey to move forward. Check back in with your *why* and your *why*. How can you measure the results of your why?

   For example, the *why* driving me to regain my health was my fatty liver diagnosis. Through my research, I discovered that ditching sugar could help me reverse this unsettling diagnosis. Eventually, this led me to the knowledge and pursuit of regulating my blood sugar, which led me to track my blood sugar. I strongly desired to lose weight, so I tracked my weight and body fat percentage on my scale.

   To help me understand the impact of sugar on my healing journey, I also began to track my food and drink consumption on the *CarbManager* app. As I learned more about living in a state of ketosis (being fueled by ketones and fat, as opposed to sugar), I tracked that too.

   Progress tracking helps you see the incremental achievements, which is highly motivating. Remember our goal-setting technique, PACT? The focus of this technique is *output*. Tracking your output provides momentum and will encourage you to keep moving forward and fixing your health based on your findings.

3. **Self-Efficacy and Positive Affirmations**. I combined these two because it's time we stop the negative and self-defeating conversations in our minds. Self-efficacy is the belief in your ability to

achieve your goals. Using positive affirmations to strengthen this belief is vital. Combined, they increase confidence in your capability, moving you to the most crucial part of your transformation journey—*take action.*

I know what runs through your mind and the negative self-talk on replay. I know because I heard and believed these thoughts for decades. "I'm a failure. Nothing I ever do is good enough. I mess up every day, so why bother? It's not fair that I can't have *that!* Might as well start again on Monday."

Stop. Breathe. Flip it around. I believe in you. I have faith in you. You are ready to reframe these immobilizing patterns. So, instead, let's try some positive affirmations to increase your self-efficacy.

Try this. "With God's help, I can win. I'm capable; I can make a good effort. My health is worth it, so I will show up every day. I choose this over that because I care for my health. I can have that wholesome and nutritious food from God's good smorgasbord! I'm enjoying every step while learning many lessons about myself."

I asked my coaching community to provide their favorite positive affirmations (and by the way, they're in the community because they believe in themselves). Would you begin to adapt affirmations like these?

"I am a beautiful daughter of the King."

"I make good choices."

"God gives me strength to overcome."

"I can do everything through Him who gives me strength." (Philippians 4:13)

You may be familiar with that often-quoted verse. Are you familiar with the context in which Paul is writing? In verses 10–12, we read that Paul is *content.* I discovered contentment in my options and my choices while God worked on my heart and changed the tune of the negative thoughts leading to destructive behavior with my approach to my health. Instead, join me in turning these thoughts to honor God in our journey. Can you learn to be content and positive in any and every situation? Whether well fed or not, whether living in plenty or want? I believe you'll enjoy living in contentment. Positive affirmations usher in peace in this process. Use them.

4. **Fear of Consequences.** Let's explore the fear of failure. No one sets out to fail, right? You didn't pick up this book thinking, "I'm ready to fail again." Nope. You picked up this book because, despite past failures, you face serious health consequences if you keep doing the same thing repeatedly with little to zero results. Hey, I've been there, done that. The idea of future health consequences related to obesity sounds dreadful. Loss of limbs, neuropathy of the extremities and retinas, immobility, kidney failure, liver failure, etc. You get the idea.

   However, in my mind, what I feared the most was sadly sitting on the sidelines of life. All my friends and family are running around, exploring new places and new mountain trails, and there I sit, pretending to read a book with a shattered heart. I hated that feeling; it was a key motivator to get me moving. Living in fear of consequences is paralyzing. Does that make sense? What consequences do you fear right now?

5. **Passion and Enthusiasm.** Flipping that fear filled my life with a new passion, song, a heart full of joy, and great enthusiasm to share this news with you! And I might add this passion God developed in me is worthy of protection. I guard my choices and steward this healing well because it's my joy and delight to serve and guide you to your freedom and greater joy. As a sister in Christ, I love you and long for you to taste and see the Lord is good. He can also fill your heart with a new passion and enthusiasm for your health. Pause and pray for God to provide this passion for you now because it's a powerful stimulus for motivation and change.

Motivational Influence

External or internal factors can influence motivation. Here are five top influences impacting my journey and coaching clients.

1. **Intrinsic Satisfaction.** Indeed, my joy increased daily as my freedom from sugar and food cravings diminished. This gift of joy filled

my heart to overflowing. I began to enjoy life in ways I never expected, which significantly motivated me to continue this lifestyle transformation. Your inherent enjoyment is vital.

2. **Perceived Control.** As I've shared, breaking up with sugar step-by-step allows us to finally experience a level of control in our food choices that we've never experienced in our years of practicing *everything in moderation.* Think about trying to moderate your sweet tooth or junk food habit. How often does restraint go out the window? Instead, busting your sugar cravings ushers in a sense of control and allows you to make better choices through your actions. You are motivated to continue these new and healthy habits when you feel in control.

3. **Values and Personal Meaning.** Have you contemplated your values regarding your health? Are you on a mission to regain your health for longevity and vitality? Yes, you have, or you wouldn't be reading these words. These values, held deeply, will motivate you to keep moving forward.

4. **Role Models and Influential Figures.** When you find a few trusted role models in your world who positively influence you to dig deep and develop healthy habits, you would be wise to remain in their sphere of influence. Of course, you must be discerning about who you follow, but an authentic and vulnerable person sharing their story to help your story will motivate you and encourage you to reach higher and passionately pursue your health goals. I would love to be one of those people in your world. Just sayin'!

5. **Emotions and Mood.** Let me leave you with the last motivational factor that will segue us into the next section of this book, "Renewing Your Mind." Hold onto your hats because confronting our journey, thoughts, and feelings will be intense. Emotions and mood will impact your motivation.

Stay positive! Remaining enthusiastic and excited about the output of your efforts will boost your motivation. Be cautious of your negative emotions and snap yourself out of a negative mood. Anxiety and stress, for example, will put a damper on your motivation and keep you stuck in the familiar place you're longing to break free from!

Before we move to the next section, I have one more question about motivation.

Is Motivation Enough?

Short answer: no. Motivation is not enough, but it should move you *to act*. Acting leads to transformation—and that, of course, is our heart's desire.

Knowing our motivation is crucial to a heart transformation. Imagine my surprise when I heard this phrase uttered during a podcast episode: "*Motivation is garbage!*"[23]

I wondered aloud, "Excuse me? What did I hear? Motivation is key to a heart transformation. This can't be right." I hit replay to hear what was just said for the context.

I listened as influencer Mel Robbins shared her life-changing formula for success. It's the title of her best-selling book, *The 5-Second Rule*. Well, it sounds like having a five-second rule could be very motivating, don't you think? Doesn't sound like garbage to me—and I've just written this whole chapter to encourage you to find motivational strategies. I needed more info and discovered a full quote on Twitter.

> "Motivation is garbage. Stop waiting to feel like it.
> Whatever it is that you want—wake up and go get it.
> With hard work, patience, and optimism,
> you can make absolutely anything happen."[24]

I find that quote very motivational, even if she is dissing motivation as a concept. The rest of it will bring about that transformation you desire. But it will take a lot of courage, do you agree? It's time to move forward into the next section of this journey—the section concerning our mind! Remember this HEART journey: *Handle Our Emotions, Examine Our Thoughts, Ask for Motivation, Run with Courage,* and *Take*

Action. Let's armor up with a shield of victory with these warrior words from King David.

Shield of Victory
You, O Lord, keep my lamp burning;
my God turns my darkness into light.
With your help I can advance against a troop;
with my God I can scale a wall.
As for God, his way is perfect:
The word of the Lord is flawless.
He is a shield for all who take refuge in him.
For who is God besides the Lord?
And who is the Rock except our God?
It is God who arms me with strength
and makes my way perfect.
He makes my feet like the feet of a deer;
he enables me to stand on the heights.
He trains my hands for battle;
my arms can bend a bow of bronze.
You give me your shield of victory,
and your right hand sustains me;
you stoop down to make me great.
You broaden the path beneath me,
so that my ankles do not turn.
—Psalm 18:28–36

Before marching forward into the emotional component, take time to get your thoughts on paper on how this journey has impacted your beliefs on restoring your physical health and your body.

A Note to Your Former Self:

A Note to Your Future Self:

Transform-Action Task:

SECTION 3: RENEWING YOUR MIND

Renew (verb): to make like new, restore to
freshness, vigor, or perfection.[25]

Do not conform any longer to the pattern of this world,
but be transformed by the renewing of your mind.
Then you will be able to test
and approve what God's will is—
his good, pleasing and perfect will.
—Romans 12:2

CHAPTER 8

FLIPPING THE MINDSET SCRIPT

I scanned the room for a seat. There were plenty of empty chairs, but where should I sit? I kept my head down and slid nonchalantly into the safest place for me. Me and my wracked emotions. Did anyone see me?

One of the greatest mysteries in my weight-loss battle is the stark difference in how I am treated in public now as a thinner woman. On some level, society tends to judge or even openly criticize the overweight. I'm sure you would agree it can be embarrassing sometimes, but perhaps it's more like a battle in the mind. Stick with me here.

I feel so out of place whenever I walk into this room. Like I'm the elephant in the room! These were the random thoughts that constantly rolled through my mind. Thoughts and emotions that kept me stuck for decades.

Of course, I'm not an elephant! Neither are you. But, boy, do these emotions and feelings well up in those circumstances. It's time to tackle what I believe to be the most challenging aspect of a successful weight-loss journey—the raging battle in our minds. This entire section on Renewing Your Mind will focus on the two critical components of a heart transformation: *H* for Handling Our Emotions and *E* for Examining Our Thoughts. I always tell my coaching clients, "This is where your hard work resides." And you've heard the age-old question and answer, "How do you eat an elephant? One bite at a time." This is a perfect strategy as we move along step-by-step in this journey.

Remember when I introduced the two *why* questions in chapter 2, "Reviewing Our Past"? It's time to get honest here and ask yourself, "*Why* did I end up here in poor health?"

I have a disclaimer. I am not a psychologist or a theologian. Throughout this book, I will offer my personal experiences and observations of the women I have coached on this challenging journey to weight-loss success.

When I am honest with myself and confront all the ugly truths, I'm led to ask the ultimate question: "Are my patterns and behaviors with food sinful?"

Go ahead and ask yourself the same question. Take your time to respond. Please journal your answer before we head any further.

All right, as a Christ-follower, I mean those of us who have made the personal decision to follow Jesus Christ, here is an important question to ask as we pursue the truth God has for each of us in our health and wellness:

"Am I fit?"

Asking that question, I'm unsure if we can confirm we are fit or at our best in our holistic health. Are we physically fit? Emotionally fit? Spiritually fit?

Would you pass muster? Is that enough? Passing muster is simply adequate or satisfactory. It's a great place to start, but are you called to something more?

I am privileged to have deep discussions with women who are longing to be free from their physical woes and worries but also can't recognize the hurdles in their emotional and spiritual health they've neglected for years. And years.

Look, I'm not judging—please don't take this personally—I have been there, done that for three decades of my adult life. And because I now know the power of God's Word, it hurts my heart when I learn from women that they rarely pick up their Bible and can't wrap their minds around their insatiable hunger from an emotional health perspective.

And dare we whisper the word gluttony in church? How often do you hear a sermon about gluttony? Come to think of it, I don't recall one while sitting in a church—so I set out to do some research.

To help you flip your mindset script, I'll begin by providing some profound food for thought. The goal here is to help you handle your emotions and examine your thoughts surrounding your food behavior. It's time to answer our second *why*.

When contemplating the word gluttony, I ask myself, "Is gluttony a sin? Am I a glutton?" Or how about the question, "What is sinful behavior regarding my relationship with food?"

"What is a sin?"

I don't have the answer to such a personal question in *your* journey, but I can answer it for myself, which I will share as we move along through this chapter's theme of allowing God to flip the mindset scripts controlling our food behaviors.

While researching how best to explain my experience with this vital question, I came across a quote from the mother of a well-known evangelist, John Wesley, the founder of the Methodist church. Susanna Wesley penned this response on sin when her son asked, "What is a sin?"

Take this rule: whatever weakens your reason, impairs the tenderness of your conscience, obscures your sense of God, or takes off your relish of spiritual things; in short, whatever increases the strength and authority of your body *over your mind*, that thing is sin to you, however innocent it may be in itself. —Susanna Wesley (Letter, June 8, 1725)[26]

Mic drop, Susanna Wesley!

This quote will help us explore the answer to our questions in our health battle and allow Scripture and God to begin the difficult work of flipping the harmful and damaging scripts running through our minds, impacting our hearts and whole health. Let's break it down by phrase.

I'll share my personal story and guide how our food behavior might fit into the wisdom from this quote. In each nugget of knowledge, I'll share the *negative* impact on our mindset while providing hope with the *positive* results of the mindset shift that can happen when we apply the strategies of living Sugar*Freed* for the glory of God.

Whatever Weakens Your Reason

Out of control. That's how I felt about my overindulgence of food when I would stuff myself into a state of misery. I recall the *negative* mindset that constantly weakened my reason: excuses, justifications, and my "I deserve this" mentality.

Acting on these emotions of entitlement would lead me to overeat until I could eat no more. Some might call this binge-eating, but I would never say that out loud. That word is scary. But as I look back, I realize how easy it is to overeat the highly palatable foods loaded with sugar and carbohydrates. It always left me weak, lacking sound reasoning around my portion choices. Sometimes, I would lie in bed at night, wondering how all that food fit into my stomach. How big is that pouch anyhow? And, of course, as I lay there, the acid reflux would cause me to choke and sit straight up in bed to catch my breath and run for the Tums.

What was I thinking? Night after night, this burning sensation in my throat should be considered unreasonable. Right?

Consider this proverb: "A man without self-control is like a city broken into and left without walls" (Proverbs 25:28 ESV).

What does this proverb have to do with our food choices? We must begin making wise and reasoned choices about our food, and to do that, we must develop self-control. Just as a city wall protects the citizens from external threats, so will our exercise of self-control equip us to make sound and reasonable food choices, helping us resist overindulgence and gain healthy control.

In "Restoring Your Body," you read many *positive* strategies to strengthen your emotional health by adopting a Sugar*Freed* way of eating. As we gradually eliminate sugar and highly refined carbs from our food choices, we physiologically and psychologically bust sugar cravings, strengthening our reason and ability to make good choices for our body, mind, and spirit. We can break free from the unhealthy food that weakens our reason.

Whatever Impairs the Tenderness of Your Conscience

I had to look up the definition of conscience to be precise. It is defined as the inner sense of what is right or wrong in one's conduct or motives, impelling one toward right action.[27]

Oh, yes. I know what it feels like to be guilty about my food behaviors.

The guilt and shame piled up and hurt my heart. We can see the *negative* impact because God does not desire us to carry the heavy weight of guilt and shame. I reflect on not just days but months and months, turning into years of negativity about my life, running through my thoughts all day, every day. And I can't forget my sensitivity to the words and actions of others; no doubt that impaired the tenderness of my conscience.

Taking responsibility for my thoughts and actions, though, I know my choices regarding my health not only hurt my heart and conscience but also my physical health, which manifested in obesity, and my spiritual health by creating a separation between my Creator and myself. Not to mention, I struggled daily with self-conscientiousness. *Me* focused, indeed.

How do we flip this mindset and start consciously living right (not wrong) for the glory of God? For a *positive* strategy, let's turn to a favorite passage that reminds me God restores and forgives whatever is impairing our consciences.

> Create in me a pure heart, O God, and *renew a steadfast spirit within me.* Do not cast me from your presence or take your Holy Spirit from me. Restore to me the joy of your salvation and grant me a willing spirit, to sustain me. (Psalm 51:10–12, emphasis mine)

What a promise! Pray through this passage if your food behaviors weigh heavy on your conscience. You can trust God in His Word to repair what you've impaired. Hallelujah!

Whatever Obscures Your Sense of God

I'm embarrassed to admit this, but when I considered quitting sugar for my health, I wrestled the following with God: "Why must I sacrifice and surrender such things when others don't have to? Why does sugar make me fat but not her? How is this even fair?"

In addition to this self-pity, other issues of my food behaviors obscured my sense of God. I'll call them obstructions—obstructions like overindulgence, negative self-talk, neglecting self-care, and idolizing food. Whoa, that's quite the list. Which obstructions do you deal with? How profound is the *negative* impact on your sense of God?

Knowing what I know now, my constant obsession and fixation on where my next meal was coming from established food as an idol in my life, and it created a fortified barrier in my relationship with God. Again, it's embarrassing to admit, but food was the central focus of my life. Even if I was physiologically addicted to sugar and carbs, I had a responsibility to dig deeper into my problem, and I did not. However, I fully believe that God had His hand over my situation and was the one to draw me to His solution.

Let's flip this obscurity with clarity from the promises of God found in Isaiah. "Forget the former things; do not dwell on the past. See, I am doing a new thing! Now it springs up; do you not perceive it? I am making a way in the desert and streams in the wasteland" (Isaiah 43:18–19).

What an encouragement to help us shift our focus from constantly dwelling on our past mistakes. It's time to embrace this new thing God is doing in your life. I love that promise, and Isaiah provides it with an exclamation point! *See, I am doing a new thing!* I hope that provides you with hope for renewal.

And here is more *positive* news. God can and will bring forth new opportunities, remove obscurities, and make a clear path for you to follow, even in this extremely challenging endeavor of weight loss.

The *way in the wilderness* and *streams in the wasteland* symbolize God's ability to provide guidance where you may be confused like me when I asked, "How is this fair?" It's time to move beyond our sinful food behavior and trust God in what He calls you to surrender and sacrifice. Do you trust God's promises and capacity to bring clarity and renewal to your journey? Even when you can't yet see the full extent of His plans, He will give you clarity over obscurity for His good plan and purpose in your healthy life. As I always remind my coaching clients, "*You show up, God shows off!*"

Whatever Takes Off Your Relish of Spiritual Things

The language is antiquated. Still, in modern language, this has a *negative* impact on your spiritual health and your appetite for spiritual matters (pun intended). Do you hunger for God's Word? Are you enthusiastic in your quiet time with the Lord? Would someone look at your spiritual walk and witness the joy of the Lord? Your struggles could be external or internal influences distracting or deterring you from a deeper connection with God.

Oh, the many things that distracted and deterred me from a deeper relationship with my Creator. The weight of the heavy chains I carried alone most definitely dulled my light. Biblical joy never crossed my mind, never settled in my heart. No wonder the decades of neglecting the promises and the path God had for me left me emotionally tired and ashamed. Perhaps in my misery, I was even afraid to show up out of fear of failure and condemnation. Again.

But let's find the shine in the *positive* steps we must take to prevent the dullness and fogginess in our minds. I have three suggestions for you to rekindle the joy in this journey.

First, *be compassionate to yourself.* I know this is hard, but did you know there is no condemnation, no blame, for you who are in Christ Jesus? Paul writes, "Therefore, there is now no condemnation for those who are in Christ Jesus" (Romans 8:1).

Second, *seek God's presence diligently.* On days when my mind wanders, and I'm prone to lose my way, I dig in deeper and sharpen my thoughts with Scripture promises like this one written by King David: "You have made known to me the path of life; you will fill me with joy in your presence, with eternal pleasures at your right hand" (Psalm 16:11). Ask the Lord to shine a light on your path, then remain in His presence daily.

Lastly, *confess and turn from the decisions clouding your mind* and dissuading you from choosing what's better for your whole health (body, mind, and spirit). I am grateful for how God drags us through and brings us to emotional and spiritual maturity. God assures us that He will forgive. "If we confess our sins, he is faithful and just and will forgive us our sins and purify us from all unrighteousness" (1 John 1:9).

In our pursuit of the renewal of our mind for the glory of God, we must remain diligent in staying centered in our spiritual walk. What step do you need today to rekindle your enthusiasm for your walk with Christ?

Whatever Increases the Strength and Authority of Your Body over Your Mind

Oh boy, here is where the rubber meets the road. I have plenty of history to confess and share to urge you to examine your food behaviors. Factors and behaviors lead to out-of-control situations in which physical impulses and bodily desires overpower our emotional and mental control.

How often do we respond to our fleshly cravings by overeating or indulging in unhealthy food and drink? Each episode gives more power to these poor decisions than your current mental and emotional capacity and self-discipline allow. The result? We are all very familiar with the yo-yo dieting cycle and patterns of self-destructive behavior, not to mention the havoc it wreaks in our minds.

Are these impulses and behaviors sinful?

Again, I can't see your heart, but I certainly know the wretchedness that resided in mine for decades that exhibited my sin.

How did I respond? Sugar binges, overeating sugar and salt cycles, and an emotional cascade of negative and defeating thoughts. I was feeding disease and hiding from God—from His purpose and calling. Considering what dulled the relish in my spiritual walk, I picture my former self as a snuffed candle, hiding a light, incapable of seeing the freedom available to me. The *negative* impact truly impacted my entire health in the following ways:

1. **Unhealthy Eating Habits:** I often felt that my body gained authority over the mind partly through the pull of those hyper-palatable foods. This led to overeating, emotional eating, secret eating, and poor dietary choices, all of which created my physical health issues. Food was how I coped.

2. **Lack of Self-Control:** For decades, I lacked this gift of the Spirit (see Galatians 5:22–23). Despite my best intentions, I did not make informed decisions or exercise self-control when my body's desires took over, making it extremely difficult to resist temptations.

3. **Emotional and Mental Health:** My struggle with obesity tremendously burdened my mental and emotional well-being. As a

result, it piled on low self-esteem, depression, and anxiety, reinforcing my unhealthy habits.

4. **Physical Health Issues:** My obesity contributed to the health problems I shared in earlier chapters. The result? Allowing my body to have authority over the mind exacerbated these health woes.

5. **Spiritual Well-Being:** For Christian women like me, obesity can affect our spiritual well-being as we struggle with feelings of guilt, shame, or a sense of disconnect from our faith due to physical health challenges (to reconnect, make sure to follow the advice given above).

To flip this around for *positive* results, we must address this issue, commit to and act on regaining control over our minds, and make informed, healthy choices for our bodies. Seeking support from your faith community, healthcare professionals, and therapists can be valuable in regaining balance between the mind and body, ultimately leading to improved overall health and well-being. As a health coach, I'd love to be part of your journey!

Let's revisit the critical verse I shared for these two sections of our body and mind. Here is your exhortation to commit.

Therefore, I urge you, brothers, in view of God's mercy, to offer your bodies as a living sacrifice, holy and pleasing to God—this is your spiritual act of worship. Do not conform to the pattern of this world, but be transformed by the renewing of your mind. Then you will be able to test and approve what God's will is—his good, pleasing and perfect will. (Romans 12:1–2)

That Thing Is Sin to You, However Innocent It May Be in Itself

"But it's not fair!"

I get it. It doesn't seem fair that your sister has always been a skinny minny, and now you're being urged to examine what might be a sin in your food behaviors and commit to making significant choices in your life.

I appreciate the admonishment, *that thing is a sin to you…*

Those behaviors (I listed above) were indeed sins to me. I was fixated and obsessed with thoughts of food, like "Where will my next delicious meal come from?" Those fixations led to sinful and impulsive behavior. As I idolized food, I now realize I was out of control!

Are they sin to you? I don't know. Only God and the Holy Spirit can provide a healthy conviction in the answer to that question.

Is eating a brownie a sin? We'd love to say no, but this is what I know. I could make brownies for my children, eat one ooey-gooey piece (seems innocent enough), and then polish off more when everyone else had gone to bed. Ugh. This left me feeling guilty and ashamed of my secret eating every time. I never thought to invite God into this battle.

In hindsight, I now realize my food behaviors were sinful and created a chasm between me and God, and I delayed my healing for decades. It was plain to see on the outside (my obese body) the severity of my struggle. It was more challenging to see the disease in my heart, mind, and soul. But recognizing that my secret eating, my obsession with food, my impulsive behavior, and my poor mood—all of which left me with a load of guilt and shame—*that thing was sin to me.*

And honestly, I was constantly convicted by my behaviors. I would never admit that to you, to my family ... or God. But I'm here now, ready to confess the *negative* consequences of polishing off one ooey-gooey brownie weighed heavy on my conscience. There's that healthy conviction. I want to share this impactful verse again. It resonates with me now, although I'm sure I glanced over it for decades. "So whether you eat or drink or whatever you do, do it all for the glory of God" (1 Corinthians 10:31).

How do we flip this around with *positive* behavior and testimonies for God's glory?

We start by sitting down with God and the Bible, praying with our hands open, seeking His guidance, and inviting Him into our struggles. This act of surrender and obedience can lead to transformation and healing. I encourage you to begin today if you haven't already started this process. It's time to address how your food behaviors align with your faith, no matter how innocent the food may be. By faith, you must begin making healthy choices to nourish your body, mind, and spiritual health. And by faith, believe this promise that Paul writes as you reconcile your food behaviors with the Lord. "Therefore, if anyone is in Christ, the new creation has come; the old has gone, the new has come" (2 Corinthians 5:17).

Hallelujah! This verse speaks to the transformative power of faith in your health journey as we reconcile and strengthen our relationship with God. This is your invitation to begin the difficult work of renewing your mind and embracing a new, more spiritually fulfilling way of living to the glory of God! How now shall we carry on?

Choose What Is Best

Now that I've invited you to contemplate, "What is a sin?" I want to leave you with a strategy for addressing this question as you work it out with God. I don't know about you, but this work of the mind and our emotional health can leave me anxious. Does it disrupt your peace?

One of the best passages to remind me of my peace and joy in Jesus is the letter Paul wrote to the Philippians. You are probably familiar with the well-loved verse in Philippians 4:7, but this entire passage provides greater peace, joy, and hope.

> Do not be anxious about anything, but in everything, by prayer and petition, with thanksgiving, present your requests to God. And the peace of God, which transcends all understanding, will guard your hearts and your minds in Christ Jesus. Finally, brothers, whatever is true, whatever is noble, whatever is right, whatever is pure, whatever is lovely, whatever is admirable—if anything is excellent or praiseworthy—think about such things. Whatever you have learned or received or heard from me, or seen in me—put it into practice. And the God of peace will be with you. (Philippians 4:6–9)

And the peace of God, which transcends all understanding, will guard your hearts and your minds in Christ Jesus. Praise God! Because I don't know about you, I need an extra measure of peace in my mind when I struggle with how God wants me to honor Him with how I steward my health.

Remember, I mentioned that flipping the mindset may be the most difficult part of this journey for you. Dealing with sin is not to be taken lightly, so I want to leave you with hope and exhortation from theologian Matthew Henry.

> A blessed change takes place in the sinner's state, when he becomes a true believer, whatever he has been. Being justified by faith he has peace with God. The holy, righteous God, cannot be at peace with a sinner, while under the guilt of sin. Justification takes away the guilt, and so makes way for peace. This is through our Lord Jesus Christ; through him as the great Peace-maker, the Mediator between God and man.[28]

Keep all of this in mind; hold it in your heart. Write down Susanna Wesley's quote in your journal for easy reference. In the next chapter, we will begin destroying destructive patterns of food behavior. Our work is hard, but dedicating your best effort and time is worth it.

A Note to Your Former Self:

A Note to Your Future Self:

Transform-Action Task:

CHAPTER 9
DESTROYING OLD
BEHAVIOR PATTERNS

In a world inundated with fad diets and failed mantras, it's time to break free from the shackles of outdated advice. You've undoubtedly received this advice repeatedly in your weight-loss efforts. And you've learned to trust it since it comes from health experts. But after years of losing your weight-loss battle, is it trustworthy? Has it taken over your thoughts and the emotions you experience in your pursuit of health? Thoughts and emotions drive behavior, and it's time we destroy the food behaviors and poor advice destroying our health, so armor up!

Ditch Dietary Dogma

"Eat less, move more," they say. *"Calories in, calories out,"* they explain—as if the human body is a formulaic input-output robot. And how about the advice that kept me bound for decades, *"Everything in moderation"*?

What if real behavior change isn't about these dreaded dietary dogmas but about the consistent small steps we take daily? In this chapter, we will debunk our pattern of relying on this dietary advice, which impacted our behaviors and kept us locked in a vicious cycle of yo-yo dieting. Write down my new advice: *Small habit changes build and deliver big results.*

You may be familiar with the idea that it takes twenty-one days to form a new habit. While that's a great place to start, it's not long enough to usher in a transformative lifestyle change. So, when I titled this chapter with the action task of *destroying old behavior patterns*, I must warn you that your work ahead will be hard. And you can't let up. Again, please repeat after me: *Small habit changes build and deliver big results.* Set your mind on building these small habits today. It's time to stop spinning your wheels.

Reflecting on eating less and moving more, my first memory is intense hunger, leading to a *hangry* state. No one likes momma in a *hangry* state. Trust me. It shines a light on how I deprived my body of the proper nourishment as I strived to lose weight. Moving more, also known as exercise, in a *hangry* state is counterproductive and leads to frustration. Again, I'm eternally grateful that my cardiologist encouraged me with the truth that weight loss is about 90 percent of what goes in your mouth and maybe 10 percent of movement and exercise. Did I mention I wanted to kiss him? He destroyed that failed mantra of *eating less and moving more* in one short conversation.

Now, don't get me wrong. Moving your body is very important, especially as we age, ladies. I encourage you to build your strength and increase your flexibility, balance, and agility, which will serve you well into the future (and prevent serious injury if you fall!). But it's time to realize that busting your behind in the gym will not deliver your weight-loss dreams. I'm living proof of this concept, as are my coaching clients. I have a perfect example of this to share with you today. Meet Heidi.

Heidi is dedicated, determined, diligent, and open to learning new ways to tackle something hard. That's how I would describe her. She's one of my best friends, whom I had the privilege of coaching past her old habits to adopt new behaviors for her health.

Sitting on the beach during our annual girl's weekend, I recall admiring her daily Zumba sessions. Here, the rest of us sat around reading books and relaxing, but Heidi would never neglect her exercise. She also excitedly spoke about her Zumba gals, the ladies on the YouTube video leading the workout. She showed me a video, and I thought, "Meh, that's not for me. I'm not that coordinated." But I encouraged Heidi to carry on—despite thinking, "You've been busting your butt for years with Zumba and your regular activity and still can't shake your little bit of excess weight."

Let me tell you, Heidi has never had a lazy bone in her body. Never. I've known her since age six, and she is always on the go! And always that person to jump up and get the physically demanding activities completed. Like building our roaring campfires.

As we approached the peri-menopausal season of life, she became frustrated with her weight and would share her frustrations with me. Over a few summers, I shared the new knowledge I discovered from my low-carb lifestyle. She'd nod, say things like, "Interesting!" and continue eating her bland salad. Looking back, I thought she was undereating, and I believe I told her a few times to "eat a steak!"

I like to plant seeds, hoping that someone will reach out to me when they reach their turning point moment. I'll never forget the day Heidi arrived at her fork in the road and reached out. I will turn this over to Heidi and let her share some of her story in her own words now.

———

Heidi Moyer—How I Danced My Way to Health by Ditching the Former Ways

I had always considered myself to be a healthy person. Whenever I felt like I was losing ground, I would exercise more! It's true; I loved my Zumba videos, walking, hiking, and biking.

However, as I approached the age of fifty, the weight crept up. It became easier to tell myself that it was good to graze all day instead of having big meals. And I liked easy. I'd come home and throw something packaged into the microwave for dinner and continue grazing into the evening on my favorite cookies, cakes, chips, dips, breakfast bars, nuts— factory foods galore!

By 2021, I felt like I had to go to bed with a full stomach; otherwise, I didn't feel quite right. I would wake up very early with a headache, and during the day, my feet would tingle, and my joints and muscles would ache. Despite my love for movement, I spent my workdays in what I describe as *swimming through clay*. I thought, "Wow, I am only in my early fifties. How is this going to feel when I'm in my seventies? This really can't be good."

During my annual physical in 2021, my doctor told me I was prediabetic. And just like Christine, I arrived at my turning point moment. That news scared me. I couldn't believe I had damaged my body like this. I thought my active lifestyle would allow me to eat what I wanted!

I started to ask questions, read literature, and learn all I could about my diagnosis. I telephoned Christine and asked her questions, especially about my morning routine and love of coffee. The first thing I do every morning is sit down to read my daily Bible lesson and have two huge cups of coffee with artificial sugar and flavored creamer. That's right. I doubled up on the sweet stuff. In her kind manner, she said, "No, the sugar has got to go!"

It was tough love, but I needed it. Without hesitation, Christine recommended I ditch sugar and starches. I immediately followed her advice and committed to God to repair what He had provided me—my body.

I adopted a new evening routine to prepare and portion my food for the next day. I ate all the food within a twelve-hour window (that's my routine of time-restricted eating) and gave up snacking, especially in those evening hours. This new habit of choosing food and packaging it up took about two weeks to feel comfortable and confident. It is now second nature; I have been doing it for two years. I will never change this method.

At the start of my commitment to a no-sugar or starch lifestyle, I lost about two pounds a week. This had never happened before in my life. I kept this up until I was pleased with my weight loss, and then I adjusted the amount of food little by little in each package to stabilize the weight loss. I tweak occasionally if I see the scale moving in the wrong direction. Unfortunately, it is never down but always up. That is always the case. I'm sure you can relate. Diligence is key once you find what works to free you from chronic disease.

Since I try to control my blood sugar spikes, my active lifestyle helps keep this in check. You will still find me taking a morning lap around the parking lot at work or running up the three flights of stairs twice daily. This is great for both your body and your mind. After eating lunch, I always go for a lunchtime walk, no matter the weather (no excuses). I'm also enjoying a fifteen-minute workout with weights at least twice weekly. I learned that using those muscles burns glucose!

In closing, at my last doctor's visit, I told my doctor that she had saved my life by telling me of my condition so that I could change my direction. She was surprised I had lost so much weight, restored a normal HbA1c, and maintained this new lifestyle for two years. She even asked me how I had done it, and I was so pleased to tell her.

I hope my story has inspired you with this fact: there is always time to make a change. Take Christine's hard-earned advice and join me in building new healthy habits today!

———

Considering I had witnessed Heidi's struggles for a few years before she received that scary diagnosis, it's easy to see how incredibly proud I am of her dedication to destroying her old food behaviors and adopting a new way of eating to reinvigorate her life. I credit her for being interested and genuinely curious about this lifestyle that worked for me. She asked insightful and interesting questions. And I know she was proud of me but couldn't see herself needing my journey or adopting my new habits. She wasn't that overweight either! Deep down, she believed dancing her brains out would lead to weight-loss victory! Right?

Wrong! I'll never forget the day she reached out to "pick my brain" even more. The day my thinnest friend was diagnosed with prediabetes. I didn't see that coming, either. But indeed, Heidi was what we call *skinny-fat*. Thin on the outside, fat on the inside. And it was her diet that did it to her. No amount of Zumba would cure this condition.

Heidi took my advice and ran with it (remember, she's very active … ha!). She showed no reluctance in making what worked for me work for her health, too. Did I mention she is a great rule follower?

Heidi's primary mission for her lifestyle change was to reverse this diagnosis of prediabetes and improve other health markers like her BMI, sleep hygiene, gut health, and joint pain and inflammation. She did not set out to lose weight, but a very nice benefit of changing what she was putting in her mouth did result in an over twenty-pound weight loss.

Now, Heidi enjoys food choices from God's good smorgasbord and will choose fruits and vegetables a little higher in sugar. Heidi can do this because her metabolism can handle these choices. When I coach, I always remind my clients to properly balance our daily carbohydrate allowance. I am extremely carbohydrate intolerant and keep my carbs under twenty grams daily. Heidi finds a healthy balance, keeping her carbs under one hundred. And just because she can afford more carbs daily doesn't mean she's grabbing a Snickers bar. Nope! She now knows the fantastic health benefits of eating from the perimeter of her grocery store.

Heidi has set herself up to age well through her diet and activity. Oh, and don't you know? You will still find Heidi dancing to that Zumba beat on a hot summer's day. That girl loves her Zumba!

Congratulations, Heidi, on destroying old food choices and behaviors that didn't serve you well and adopting the Sugar*Freed* lifestyle. Let's dance to the freedom song!

Fuzzy Math

I know Heidi was greatly relieved to ditch the dietary advice of *calories in, calories out* because she hates math! And like me, she enjoys understanding how a formula such as calories in being less than calories out would function. It's a mystery to me when you stop to consider the nutritional value of one hundred calories of candy versus one hundred calories of nutrient-rich foods like steak and eggs. It's time to stop calculating how many minutes on the treadmill will help you burn off that Snickers bar. The human body is much more complex than this simple *calories in, calories out* formula.

Weight loss is a balance of many factors, mostly your hormones. What impacts your hormone health? Factors like what you put in your mouth, your sleep hygiene, your stress level, and your activity. When someone can show me a complex math formula to include all these factors, I'd love to test it out because I love math. It's never going to happen, though. So, let's kick this confusing, mathematically impossible advice to the curb by ditching our sugar!

Moderation Misnomer

Next, we have the advice that kept me chained in my sugar and food addiction for decades: *Everything in moderation.* In full transparency, I know this mantra permitted me to indulge in everything I should have avoided for my health. And not just indulge but overindulge ... because when it comes to eating sugar and carbohydrates, it is nearly impossible to hit the shut-off switch! Recall that sugar and refined carbs are highly addictive and created in the factory to be hyper-palatable. Making you run back for more. And more. And more. So much for moderation.

It's painful to admit how this behavior contributed to my sinful choices of running to food for comfort, but indeed, this behavior kept me out of control for years. Refer to the previous chapter, "Flipping the Mindset Script," to contemplate if advice like *everything in moderation* leads you astray. It's worth repeating Susanna Wesley's quote:

> Take this rule: whatever weakens your reason, impairs the tenderness of your conscience, obscures your sense of God, or takes off your relish of spiritual things; in short, whatever increases the strength and authority of your body *over your mind*, that thing is sin to you, however innocent it may be in itself. — Susanna Wesley (Letter, June 8, 1725)[29]

Relying on man-dictated dietary advice neglects the proper nourishment of our soul. It clouded my thoughts and emotions when I continually felt like a failure. When I constantly believed I was a failure, nothing felt meaningful in life. Those thoughts and emotions led me to destructive behaviors in my health. How about you? What thoughts and emotions keep you in repetitive behavior, destroying your health?

Freedom from Failed Advice

It will take some dedication to hop over these ingrained dietary mantras. We must play some mental gymnastics to rework our patterns of behavior. So, if we can't rely on this dietary advice we grew up on, what shall we rely on? Praise God that He gives us the mental capacity to handle our emotions and examine our thoughts to change our behaviors in our heart transformation journey. As we ask the Lord for motivation to do just that, we can entrust this courageous journey to Him and be spurred to act, and let's act fast!

As I write this chapter, I'm wrapping up another year and reflecting on my word of the year—*steadfast*. And I find another promise in Isaiah to increase our trust in the Lord. "You will keep in perfect peace him whose mind is *steadfast*, because he trusts in you. Trust in the Lord forever, for the Lord, the Lord, is the rock eternal" (Isaiah 26:3, emphasis mine).

Let's cling to this promise from God's Word as we embark on this transformation journey. Quitting sugar, refined carbs, and factory food will require a complete lifestyle transformation when you choose your health over a future of chronic disease. Busting old habits is hard, as you can imagine. I'm convinced you're reading this book because God instilled something in your heart to make this significant change in your life. Changing behavior is difficult but doable! For starters, let's not dwell on the past as we now see how the old dietary advice does not serve what we need for a lasting weight-loss victory. Trust God right now. He is doing something new in your health and wellness. Remember this: "You show up, God shows off!"

Keep this saying in mind when you are feeling stuck, hanging on by a thread, or falling completely off the rails. A wise woman reminded me the other day, *"Steadfast does not mean perfection!"* Phew! What a relief. Repeat it with me: Steadfast does not mean perfection.

I'm grateful that ditching sugar certainly makes losing weight easier. Just wait until you reach the day when you realize you are no longer craving sugar. I still consider it a miracle, and you will, too.

I am confident that God makes a way for us to find a healthy relationship with food for our future health. Given our human nature, our behaviors will determine our outcome. Let's return to my favorite verse regarding the heart of this matter. King David writes, "You have filled my heart with greater joy than when their grain and new wine abound" (Psalm 4:7). And knowing that God looks at the heart more than outward appearance (as opposed to man's view), let's define the heart.

From reading about the Hebrew word for heart, *leb*, or *lebib*, in the Strong's Concordance[30], we learn the term *heart* is more than just an organ that pumps blood. Indeed, being so uniquely created by God, He knits our hearts lovingly and compassionately to include characteristics of care, courage, friendliness, brokenness, and many emotions. The heart is the core of feelings, will, and intellect, portraying a versatile center associated with considerations and consent. All of which prompts us to act! It's a matter of the heart to choose healthy or hardened behaviors for our whole health—in body, mind, and spirit. The heart is the epicenter of all we say, do, think, and behave in life. I coach women to prepare for a heart transformation above all else in their health and healing journey. Our daily habits cannot change until we make this connection.

Don't run! I know your heart may be broken or shattered after all it's been through in your health endeavors, so take a breath. Please don't be overwhelmed; lean into God's grace and mercy, and He will make a way.

Psychologists say it takes twenty-one days to build new habits. You've heard me say that's not enough. It's a great place to start because, as I said, and repeat after me, "*Small habit changes build to deliver big results.*" We must begin somewhere. Let's start small, if needed.

Starting small, not biting off more than you can chew, will set you up for success. Here are four ideas you can jot down and implement over the next few weeks:

1. **Start small.** Recall my day one of quitting sugar. I gave up flavored coffee creamer (and the coffee, too). After surviving a few days (yes, it's possible to live without coffee), I chose my next small step: avoiding all the candy around my office. Then, I turned down the cakes, pies, brownies, and cookies that appeared daily in the office. Then, I began reading labels, searching for sugar and hidden sugars in processed food. And so on. Let me ask, "What is the one food or drink loaded with sugar you can live without today? And tomorrow?" Build from those daily wins.

2. **Have a plan.** My objective was to reverse fatty liver disease. I began by reverse engineering this momentous goal in the step-by-step plan I committed to when I started small. Write down every goal you long to achieve. Try to be specific. For example, if you want to incorporate exercise into your daily routine, what days and times of your week will you fit this in? Be sure to examine how realistic your plan is. Too big? Head back to tip number one to start small. Post your plan where you will see it daily.

3. **Change one behavior at a time.** We didn't get into an unhealthy mess overnight. Our destructive behaviors developed over time, so give yourself grace while adopting these new healthy behaviors. One important lesson I learned in coaching is that while I challenged women to a twenty-one-day quitting sugar boot camp, they can come out of the gate gang-busters, but a lasting lifestyle transformation takes time. Most psychologists suggest a ninety-day

commitment to these changes will likely stick. I've also observed the women I coach begin gaining their victory within a minimum of ninety days with *The* Sugar*Freed Me Weight-Loss Solution* program; I see a big difference in their results if they just stick with it. They are more dedicated and set up to succeed in a step-by-step plan to change behavior, jumping over one hurdle at a time. Ninety days is just the beginning when you consider this lifestyle change.

4. **Find support and accountability.** First, you must show up for yourself, but I guarantee that once you share your commitment and determination to make these changes, having a buddy or a coach will increase your motivation and dedication. It's my passion to support and coach women in this journey. And I've witnessed how life-changing a community of women who get you can add to your success. I'm also a huge advocate of mental health therapy for women who struggle with trauma impacting their weight-loss efforts. Don't neglect the importance of support and accountability in changing your behavior for a healthy outcome.

As you can imagine, this process is complex, but I will testify all day long from my own story and through stories like Heidi's—*you can destroy unhealthy food behaviors.* And as you work it out daily, you will soon realize you can leave those past failures behind. I'll talk about the weight of our soon-to-be past failures more in the next chapter.

A Note to Your Former Self:

A Note to Your Future Self:

Transform-Action Task:

CHAPTER 10

LEAVING FAILURES BEHIND

■ ■ ■

And here we are—time to talk about the heaviest weight we carry. And no, I'm not referring to our body fat mass. This heavy weight is *guilt and shame.* Would you agree that we are experts at dragging this around? Decades for me. How long for you?

We need to start leaving failures behind to drop this guilt and shame. That implies a drastic change, but you're worth the effort. Don't forget that this drastic overall change is a change of heart that requires motivation. Are you motivated to leave your failures behind? By now, you have read how detrimental sugar and junk food are to your whole health. You're ready! I assure you that you are prepared to leave the failed or victim mindset behind.

Let's revisit my favorite motivational quote posted in front of my face in the many places I spent time. My office, breakroom at work, kitchen, bathroom, writing space … it was in my face every day. *"You can't go back and change the beginning, but you can start where you are and change the ending."* Jot that down. Now, stick it everywhere. This will be key to dropping the heavy weight of guilt and shame.

Given that this battle is essential to our victory, let's revisit Psalm 51 and seek the Lord for help. I turn to Psalm 51 often, especially when those niggling thoughts of my past failures try to win their battle in my day. On days we barely stand up under the weight of this guilt and shame, we need sustenance from God.

Create in me a pure heart, O God, and renew a steadfast spirit within me. Do not cast me from your presence or take your Holy

Spirit from me. Restore to me the joy of your salvation and *grant me a willing spirit, to sustain me.* (Psalm 51:10–12, emphasis mine)

If we want to win our battle for a future of good health, we need to lean on David's plea. I don't know about you, but I don't see room for the weight of guilt and shame when we are dedicated to God purifying our hearts.

So, why do we carry this heavy weight of guilt and shame? Why isn't it easy to dump this extra load? It can be so unbearable. And if you're anything like me, decades of failures never let it ease up. So, it piled up. This extra load hurts our hearts. Does that sound right to you?

To be clear, let's define guilt and shame.

Guilt (noun): the state of one who has committed an offense especially consciously; feelings of deserving blame, especially for imagined offenses or from a sense of inadequacy; a feeling of deserving blame for offenses.[31]

Shame (noun): a painful emotion caused by consciousness of guilt, shortcoming, or impropriety; a condition of humiliating disgrace or disrepute; something to be regretted.[32]

Wow, those definitions resonate with me. Thinking back on my battle with guilt and shame, I know the following is true:

- Guilt says: "I consciously made poor food choices daily. I always chastised myself for these choices."
- Guilt says: "I constantly felt inadequate in every move I made."
- Guilt says: "Self-consciousness plagued my mind daily, and thoughts of 'What do others think of me?' never relented."
- Guilt says: "I deserved all the negative consequences of my choices."
- Shame says: "Painful emotions plagued my heart, mind, and soul. *Those conscious choices of poor food stuffed the emotions down.*"
- Shame says: "I regretted those choices."
- Shame says: "I am wholly and solely to blame."

Don't miss this: *Those conscious choices of poor food stuffed the emotions down.* Can you observe the vicious cycle of guilt and shame leading us over and over to turn to food to quiet our emotions? It's hard, I know. Primarily reflecting on my daily routine of starting over again, day in and day out. Or especially when every Monday rolled around. Friend, we must stomp on the *starting-over-every-Monday mentality*—it creates a pattern of failure as we make excuses for our choices.

Do you think the Lord wants us to carry this heavy weight of guilt and shame? Absolutely not! Throughout His Word, God invites us to transfer this weight to Him. He will handle it. How can we be sure of this? Let's explore how to leave failures behind and begin to heal our hearts from guilt and shame through the ministry of Jesus. Many stories in the New Testament show His caring and compassionate heart toward women who carried guilt and shame. One of my favorites in Luke 7 is the story of the sinful woman and her alabaster jar. I invite you to read Luke 7:36–50 for the full story before reading my explanation.

Let's set the scene. In the home of a Pharisee named Simon, we see a crowd, including Jesus, reclining around a table for a meal. And behind Jesus, *sitting against the wall*, we find a sinful woman, a prostitute, at the feet of Jesus. What was a sinful woman doing in the home of a respected Pharisee? And while he was hosting Jesus?

I wrote about this scene in chapter seven of my Advent devotional, *Seeking Joy through the Gospel of Luke*, and just this year, I learned important lessons about why this woman was *sitting against the wall* and the heart of the why and how Jesus treated her in this moment.

I gleaned a new richness from this passage through cultural Bible expert Kristi McLelland in her Bible study *Jesus and Women*. The Pharisees wanted to keep this woman down, yet Jesus was about to flip this scene around. Keeping in mind this woman's sinful choices, Simon, the host, thought to himself, "If this man were a prophet, he would know who is touching him and what kind of woman she is—that she is a sinner" (Luke 7:39). To which Jesus replied, "Simon, I have something to tell you" (Luke 7:40). Jesus then went on to explain through an illustration God's purpose and plan for dealing with guilt and shame.

Kristi uses examples from Scripture to explain the biblical concept of justice and righteousness to help us understand our typical Westernized cultural view of guilt and shame. As Westerners, we often think of guilt and shame as *right and wrong*. We make wrong choices; we carry the shame. We deserve whatever *justice* we put upon ourselves.

The Hebrew words for justice and righteousness are *mishpat* and *tzedakah*. Understanding the biblical meaning of these words is essential as we learn to leave our failures behind. I believe you are about to let out a massive sigh of relief when you understand God's heart of justice and righteousness over our sins. Here is an explanation of each word from Kristi.

Mishpat: Translated most often as "justice," the Hebrew word *mishpat* serves a special function in the economy of God. Since God advocates for the poor and the oppressed, especially widows and orphans, He expects His followers to do the same. At its core, *mishpat* isn't so much a question of innocence and guilt as much as honor and shame. To bring justice to the world, God exalts the humble by raising them to honor and covering their shame. Tied closely to the word *tzedakah*, or "righteousness," *mishpat* deals with punishment for wrongdoing, but it is also concerned about equal rights for all—rich and poor, female and male, foreigner and native-born.[33]

Tzedakah: means "righteousness" and so much more. Placed within the realm of relationships, *tzedakah* prompts us to make things right through generosity. Another translation for this word could easily be "mercy." In fact, in the first-century world, giving to the poor was seen as an act of righteousness (see Matthew 6:1–4). By not sharing generously, one violates the very justice, will, and command of God. *Tzedakah* is not optional in God's economy.[34]

Let's go back to the story of this sinful woman in Luke 7. Here is a woman surrendering her heart at the feet of Jesus. She showed up boldly, with perhaps a priceless gift in her possession, and she pours it all out at the feet of Jesus. Sit in this space for a moment. To move forward in your journey, ask yourself, "What priceless possession will I bring to surrender and sacrifice at the feet of Jesus?"

And most importantly, can you leave it there? Will you stop snatching it back up and carrying this heavy weight of guilt and shame?

Notice her tears and her kissing of His feet. Imagine the emotional release of the heavy burden she carried on her heart. Her heart is transforming for a future as a dedicated Christ-follower. But how will she release the guilt and shame of her sin? Jesus, that's how. Kristi writes these words to encourage you to drop this guilt and shame. Jesus wants to take them off your head, hands, and heart.

Jesus brought justice and righteousness to women in the first-century world. He generously lifted them up out of their shame and restored their honor. Jesus did not come to turn things upside down. Jesus came to turn things right side up.[35]

Read that again. Jesus did not come to banish that woman to the back of the room. No, quite the opposite. Jesus admonished Simon the Pharisee for his lack of cultural hospitality... "You did not give me any water, a kiss, some oil for my head... " but this sinful woman went above and beyond in adoring her Savior with all that and more.

Jesus saw her heart. In this moment, Jesus removed her guilt and shame and restored her honor. As she departed, He generously offered her this blessing: "Your faith has saved you; go in peace" (Luke 7:50).

Do you have faith like this woman? Do you have the faith to stand up, walk into a space where you feel like you would lack honor because of your past, and lift your gaze to Jesus? Friend, *He came to set you free!* Can't you see? God's meaning of justice and righteousness means we can move forward and leave our years of guilt and shame behind us. And we can also not have a care in the world about what the Pharisees of our day think, see, or do!

Will you find hope in my story about hearing from Dr. Fung when he uttered this short encouragement that sparks a new hope? "This is not your fault." The poor advice we received for decades ushered in guilt and shame. Does it cause you to talk poorly about yourself, too? Yes? Yeah, it did for me, too. So now what do we do?

Reflecting on Luke 7, I wrote the following in my devotional:

"The little voice in our heads loves to tell us we can't do hard things, but we can." It is simple to say, I know, I know. But hard to do. You can do it; I have faith in you.

You Can Do Hard Things

Why is it so difficult to believe we can do hard things? For me, those years of failures were my underlying fear. And lack of support. This is not to say that those closest to me didn't care about my situation; *I never freely shared with them the depths of my despair.* I hid the immense sorrow I felt. I swept the many shattered pieces of my broken heart under the mask of my fake persona. Ladies, I never even shared this pain honestly with my husband. First, he never gave me the impression that he loved me less in my condition (praise God). It was more like the elephant in the room. A sensitive topic we rarely discussed. Thinking back, I regret all those years of what I put my family through with my moodiness and lack of joy—but thankfully, I now focus on thinking forward. We learn a lot from our history, do we not?

When I gasped for air on the side of that mountain and begged God to help me feel better, I shudder to think how I might have responded had He whispered, "You're about to do the hardest thing ever and face the biggest trial in your life during this transformation." In my exhaustion, I probably would have muttered, "Pass. I'm so tired." All I can say is that when God has you right where He wants you to change your life, you better hold on tight and learn to let go.

No, I'm not contradicting myself!

You'll need to grasp tight to Jesus. Grasp tight to His garment. Remain sheltered under the protection of His wings. Read this beautiful promise from the last book of the Old Testament. A promise before God was silent for four hundred years until the birth of Jesus! "But for you who revere my name, the sun of righteousness will rise with healing in its wings. And you will go out and leap like calves released from the stall" (Malachi 4:2).

Now, fast forward four hundred years to the incarnate Jesus and His healing ministry on earth. I see the fulfillment of healing promises in a favorite story in Luke 8. In this chapter, a woman with a long-standing bleeding disorder exhibits great faith by grabbing the hem of Jesus's garment—the place where she found healing. As Jesus inquired, "Who touched me?" (Luke 8:45), the woman fell at His feet, trembling in fear, and confessed it was her.

Considering her guilt and her shame from a dozen years of living unclean (in those days, a bleeding disorder classified her as unclean, ostracizing her from community and fellowship), this woman took bold action. She stepped out with tremendous courage for her healing. Are you in a desperate place and need to do the same?

Keep in mind that although this may not be entirely our fault, it's our problem and our responsibility to take action to change our situation. We need to be diligent about leaving our failures behind in the process. It's the key to renewing our minds and improving our emotional health. I've done the work and now have the privilege to coach so many women through this tough part of their journey. So, it's my pleasure to introduce you to my client, Dee, who puts in the hard work daily, and with her gift of mercy, I believe her story will resonate with you.

———

Dee's Story—Releasing a History of Guilt and Shame

Inch by inch, I propelled myself forward with each raspy breath. I told myself, "Keep moving forward." My goal lay before me; I was nearly there.

Was I heading up some mountain peak, perhaps trekking around the globe? Or walking or hiking to a milestone? No! My destination was the bathroom!

Twenty-five feet. It felt like a thousand. I had been despondent over the way my health had taken such a turn for the worse. Having multiple autoimmune diseases, I felt not only despair but like a walking dictionary of medical terms. Daily, I lived in pain, almost too much to bear.

I would cry out to God with all my heart and ask Him to help me change the trajectory of my health. My weight had skyrocketed; I trembled at the number on the scale and felt utter despair. Was there no hope for me?

Hear my prayer, O Lord; let my cry for help come to you.
—Psalm 102:1

I prayed and prayed and tried to do everything within my power. I was determined to change my health to the best of my abilities. I asked myself, "How's that working for you?" I mean, in all seriousness, how had all the years of dieting, starting at the age of ten with a liquid diet, to *Weight Watchers* so many times I can't even remember, to Tops, Atkins, the cabbage soup diet, and so on ever help? I lost some weight with each attempt but would regain it all and then some.

I am known as a "foodie." I grew up in a restaurant, so if I wanted to see my daddy, I would have to be there. My father was a self-taught culinary giant; he would deftly turn flour, lard, salt, and water into the most luscious creations. One of my sweetest memories is standing on a bucket beside him while he feverishly created dozens of pie crusts. At the same time, I worked on a tiny piece of dough, patting it and rolling it while he taught me the intricacies of a tender, flaky crust.

Food was something we did, who we were, our identity. It was as deeply embedded within me as if it had always been part of my original DNA, and in a way, it was. Our family and all the relatives talked about food, baking, cooking, and marrying others who had restaurants. We were "My Big Fat Greek Wedding" long before the movie existed!

As an award-winning cook and baker, how could I break the chains and bondage of a mindset that constantly planned the next meal or created the next dessert? How could I ever start one more diet when I had failed every time? I had given up. I had accepted my fate as I slowly shuffled inch by inch, aided by a walker, those twenty-five endless feet to the bathroom again. Hot tears rolled down my swollen face.

I waited patiently for the Lord; he turned to me and heard my cry.
He lifted me out of the slimy pit, out of the mud and mire;
he set my feet on a rock and gave me a firm place to stand.
—Psalm 40:1–2

Then I met Christine. This effervescent, beautiful, knowledgeable soul who wanted to share what God had taught her, what He had done in her life, and how she knew something I didn't know. *There is freedom available over my food battles*! She was a living testimony to the truth that Jesus is the answer; being sugar-free was the cure. She sparked hope.

She invited me to join her in *The SugarFreed Me Weight-Loss Solution* program. She guided the way through her program, built by faith and on a foundation of faith, to learn to live free from the bondage of sugar and what it does to our bodies, minds, hearts, and souls. I told myself, "I can do this for thirteen weeks, and then I can go back to eating sugar, just in time for Christmas and all the glorious baking I'd do again!"

But wait … something happened. As I jumped in headfirst, God flipped something in my heart. And for the first time in years, I was determined to do it. And I did.

What I learned pricked my heart and my mind! How did I not know that carbs equal sugar and sugar destroys our health? I learned, I soaked it in, I grew. I went back to the Word daily. I prayed, and this time, I didn't cry hot, bitter tears for God not healing me. I took the initiative and said, "Yes, Lord, I can do this in your strength! You have a new way for me, not for a mere thirteen weeks, but you have shown me the path of freedom and allowed me to walk in it! Hallelujah!"

There is indeed freedom. The voices in my head no longer subjugate me to their constant chatter. I no longer feel enslaved, bound by the chains of sugar addiction and all that goes with it. The self-loathing, the words of self-deprecation, are gone. He has indeed created me in His image beautifully. And this day, this very moment, He has allowed me to change the future trajectory of my life by making wise and life-giving choices today for as long as He gives me breath.

The anchor and chains of shame and guilt over food are gone. However long the journey may be, I'm pleased to take each step inch by inch to bring me closer to my goal and the joy of being all I can be for Christ as I live Sugar*Freed*!"

———

Thank you, Dee! Are you ready to join Dee in leaving those anchors of guilt and shame behind? It's been my pleasure to watch Dee move through the process of leaving her past failures in the dust for over a year now. She epitomizes the woman ready to rise and face her daily, step-by-step, and often minute-by-minute food behavior challenges. Let's all cheer on Dee and her weight-loss victory!

Now, it's your turn. My friend, it's time to confront the weight of guilt and shame dragging you down. Can you see that Jesus came to set you free from this burden? Remember, *His* yoke is easy, and *His* burden is light. He would never pile on the overwhelming pain of guilt and shame. Please take my word for it … you can't climb mountains carrying heavy chains! Join me in this climb; leave your failures behind. Next, I'm excited to share the steps to busting your cravings to make climbing your mountains doable and enjoyable. Let's go!

A Note to Your Former Self:

A Note to Your Future Self:

Transform-Action Task:

Chapter 11

Controlling Cravings

■ ■ ■

We are back to the *it* and the *what* of our plethora of health woes—*Cravings.* In chapter 3, "Craving All the Wrong Things," I shared the physiological reasons we crave sugar and highly palatable food. There is so much more about cravings—deep and soul-wrenching work to explore the cravings of our mind. Oh, friend, if I had a magic formula for the mind, this could be a concise chapter. But alas, I do not, so prepare for intense work. Let's find guidance in God's Word, starting with a meaningful passage to explore the inner workings of the heart and mind regarding cravings. One must do the work deep within the heart to renew the mind.

When I began picking up my Bible daily, one of the first books I studied was Ephesians. Paul wrote this now favorite book of mine to the church in Ephesus to help believers understand God's eternal purpose and grace. This message is for you and me to renew our minds. And our hearts, bodies, and spirits. This book profoundly transformed my mind and relationship with God, so I'm excited to share the impact it had on me with you.

Ephesians 2 gives us a solid strategy. Paul addresses our health by examining *where we've been, where we are, and where we long to be.* When I read this chapter with new eyes, an open mind, and a willing heart—it rocked my world! And I know through my experience in coaching people like you that this will rock your world and provide great encouragement as you renew your mind with Christ.

Reflecting on my past behaviors pains me; my mind will carry the memories of the heavy weight of guilt and shame. I'm sure you understand.

When we suffer defeat repeatedly with our weight-loss efforts, it leaves battle scars—not only in disease but also in our minds! But reflect, we must. We've all been there, so take a deep breath, grab your journal, and let's get real.

Where We've Been

Let's turn to the first section of Ephesians 2 for clarity to see if we can identify what rattles through our minds as we pursue our health for God's glory. This chapter opened my eyes and ears to what the Lord asked of me in caring for my whole health.

> As for you, you were dead in your transgressions and sins, in which you used to live when you followed the ways of this world and of the ruler of the kingdom of the air, the spirit who is now at work in those who are disobedient. All of us also lived among them at one time, *gratifying the cravings of our sinful nature and following its desires and thoughts*. Like the rest, we were by nature objects of wrath. (Ephesians 2:1–3, emphasis mine)

Whoa. I'll begin with the ugly truth. I, indeed, was gratifying my cravings, the cravings of my flesh, through my thoughts and desires as I made food an obsession in my life. Food was my idol. I craved food, not just in the physiological way (which, again, is not wholly our fault due to the design of our modern junk food loaded with hyper-palatable sugar and fake oils), but in a way that I believe put an enormous chasm in my relationship with God. I was disobedient to His Word—evidenced by the truth that I rarely picked up my Bible for personal devotion. I was, by human nature, an object of wrath. That's my ugly truth.

That word *cravings* jumped off the page when I read this chapter for the first time in my new study. I knew by that time I was on a journey to bust my sugar cravings through my physical choices and a new understanding of what sugar did to my brain and my overall health. But what Paul writes about here concerning *cravings* took me much deeper into my healing journey. Examining my thoughts, handling my emotions, and my *feelings* ... whoa, whoa, whoa, my *feelings* (sing with me now) is where the rubber meets the road, so to speak. This means it's time to act.

Do you see all those components of the heart transformation? It's all there. And let me tell you, it's no small feat to defeat *the cravings of our sinful nature* when it's difficult even to identify what they are! Sharing my sinful depravity goes deep, and it isn't very comfortable. But I'll do my best to explain. In speaking God's message, I have learned to be comfortable with being uncomfortable. So I ask you again: *Can you be comfortable being uncomfortable?*

"I filled the nooks and crannies, the holes in my soul, while satisfying my cravings. The problem is, I craved all the wrong things." I share this in my testimony message.

And I testify that I believe God created us to crave. We were *made to crave*. Knowing God created me to crave helped me sort out my relationship with cravings.

Remember when I explained that our bodies crave essential nutrients and minerals (like salt)? Again, God created us to crave.

Not only was I craving sugar physiologically (for another dopamine hit on my brain), but I used food as comfort when I was feeling gloomy. Or glad! Food, especially junk food loaded with carbs, was my medication of choice to satisfy the cravings of thoughts and desires—all the ideas in my mind.

This is not an excuse to defend myself, but I didn't understand how God calls us to care for our health because I never read His Word. And even if I read His Word, it wasn't to change my heart toward my relationship with food! I would never utter to you or anyone that I idolized food. And gluttony! Bah, no one wants to talk about that. My history sounds so depraved because it was, and I must testify to all of it now. We will talk more about gluttony soon, but first, I want to show you God's grace in your life.

For thirty years, I lived in depravity, craving all the wrong things. *But God.* His grace and mercy showed me a way out, a way forward. He completely flipped the cravings of my life. Which brings me to where I am today and where I want you to join me.

Where We Are

You're here, which tells me the Holy Spirit prompted you to pick up this book through what I call *healthy conviction*. Or perhaps you've been following my story for a while now. Something intrigued you and caused you to *act*. You're ready to pursue your health for the glory of God and address your food behaviors and relationship with the Lord. Trust me, the reason you picked up this book is all about God. I'm just a willing vessel to guide you.

When I started writing this book in 2018, I wanted to shout from the mountaintop, "Come and see all the Lord has done for me." Don't get me wrong! It was exciting and worthy to share, but it was very shallow.

Would it surprise you that I've pushed back on God by sharing this book's emotional and spiritual messages? Really, Lord? I'm nice. I'm full of joy—why do I get to deliver hard truths? The answer lies in the number of years this book has been in process.

What a process. Has it been perfected? Oh, no! But I set out to write this long letter to you in 2018 when I was living on cloud nine, celebrating my weight-loss victory and enjoying my adult life more than I ever imagined. And I wanted you to join me there with rainbows, unicorns, and living the fairy tale. It's now 2025 (seven years in the making!), and I've been through some stuff. Some desperately hard stuff. Including a courtroom trial with billion-dollar insurance lawyers questioning my integrity and attempting to destroy my family, sabotage the care that my loved one desperately needs, and shake my faith. *But God.* He parked me *where I have been* to share these lessons with you all these years. By the way, the story about the courtroom trial is a story for another book, another day.

It's been a long season for me to be *where I am*, where God placed me, to articulate the full measure of grace He mercifully gives to each of us. Read this truth in the following few verses of Ephesians 2 to see for yourself.

But because of his great love for us, God, who is rich in mercy, made us alive with Christ even when we were dead in transgressions—it is by grace you have been saved. (Ephesians 2:4–5)

Christ makes us alive! Saved by grace through abundant mercy!

If that isn't some miracle, I don't know what is. Let's make it our goal to live alive in Christ. Do you see the way out? Do you see that God can and will flip the cravings of your life when you lean on Him to triumph over your transgressions? Over temptations. Through trials. At the same time, facing the storms of life. And even in seasons of great suffering—God can keep you alive in Christ in the battle for your good health for His good glory. Don't forget that last part.

Where I am in these years since I've surrendered my health and wellness to God could have easily put me back where I used to be. Had I not experienced His freedom and His greater joy in my heart—I shudder to think of myself satisfying the cravings of my very hurt heart due to suffering. I could have easily eaten my feelings back into morbid obesity. That was my previous pattern of behavior in my weight-loss rollercoaster.

Where am I now? By God's grace and mercy, I am living the Sugar-*Freed* life and maintaining a healthy weight, free from chronic disease that was robbing my joy in living. I no longer cave to my emotional cravings because of the glorious gift of self-control and all these years of picking up my Bible daily and trusting God with my whole heart for my body, mind, and spirit.

I share this to remind you that this journey must become your lifestyle. Your new choices and a surrendered heart will lead to freedom! Tremendous effort is required to control your physical and emotional cravings for sugar and junk food, but I implore you to pursue hard after God's grace and mercy. Ask Him right now to set you free. Ask Him to make you alive in Christ right now and for the rest of your life concerning the health of your body, mind, and spirit. Think of your future self. I love to think of my home in heaven. It's where I long to be—how about you?

Where We Long to Be

Let me guess, you long to be free from irrational and emotional food cravings, long to be healthy, long for more energy to get through the day, long to be thin, long to fit into those jeans in the back of your closet, and long to stop the obsessive and fixated thoughts about sugar and junk food. I could go on and on, but you get the idea. We all long, we all crave, for something. But let me ask you this. Do you long for a surrendered heart transformation? Are you willing to sacrifice and let God flip your life's cravings?

Because He can. Let's lift our gaze heavenward.

And God raised us up with Christ and seated us with him in the heavenly realms in Christ Jesus, in order that in the coming ages he might show the incomparable riches of his grace, expressed in his kindness to us in Christ Jesus. For it is by grace you have been saved, through faith—and this not from yourselves, it is the gift of God—not by works, so that no one can boast. For we are God's workmanship, created in Christ Jesus to do good works, which God prepared in advance for us to do. (Ephesians 2:6–10, emphasis mine)

Made alive and seated with Christ! Imagine the good smorgasbord at that table. Friend, God, through His grace and mercy, invites you to this table today (and every day)!

For the first time in my adult life, I felt welcomed and had a seat at a table—and Jesus was saving it for me. He's saving it for you, too. I've shared the dread I experienced in my self-consciousness when I walked into a room. We can also break free from that. I don't care, I don't care, *I don't care* what man thinks as long as my heart remains steadfast in chasing after what God cares about.

It's honestly taken a lot of emotional heart work to not care what people think. And what I thought they were thinking has been completely flipped. These are the thoughts I used to have:

"Ugh. I know what they're thinking. I'm obese and overindulging on all the potluck goodies." I was.

"She should eat a salad, not the deep-dish pizza." I know.

Oh, and how about this one … "She's so pretty. If only she could lose the weight."

Here is a reminder, my friend, before I go on. "Man looks at the outward appearance, but the LORD looks at the heart" (1 Samuel 16:7). I never understood that because I never studied Scripture in depth to learn the heart of God. So, no matter what those people thought about me when

I walked into an event, it shouldn't have made me feel excluded in God's eyes. Well, hindsight is always 20/20. But this is an essential lesson for you now. No matter if you are morbidly obese or need to lose only ten pounds, as a Christ-follower, there is a seat for you in the heavenly realms at His table. Let's continue with how God flipped all those negative thoughts.

Now, this could be awkward except for the transformation of my heart. Remember I said I have learned to be comfortable with being uncomfortable? I could shy away and stay home now with thoughts like this:

"No one wants me in the room because I will make them feel guilty about eating the cake, the cookies, all the things I don't eat."

"I bet they think I'm judging them."

If you truly know me personally, this is the furthest thought from my mind and heart. If you think I'm uncomfortably judging or condemning you, you are wrong.

But what I will do, and I'm called to do concerning your health, is respond to your questions, engage in conversation, and encourage you to choose wisely when God opens those doors of communication. And trust me, He will, and He does in ways I never imagined.

Everything I share is from a foundation of faith. Faith is one of my spiritual gifts (along with exhortation). First and foremost, God is faithful. God is faithful and will help you deal with your out-of-control cravings. He can flip your physical cravings and your psychological cravings. Just watch. You must be faithful to respond to the healthy conviction the Holy Spirit puts on your heart. And I became a Christian health coach because I believe in you to do the hard things.

"But how, Christine? How? I've tried and failed so many times—I'm on the edge of accepting I'll be fat for life." Hey, I hear you. Trust me. I thought that, too. And again, this will not be easy. I'm here to help you in every way possible.

But I can't do it for you. You must take action and responsibility for your health. What if you don't act? Well, besides the apparent misery of living with chronic disease (like the loss of limbs that disturbed my thoughts...), not acting may be a sin of omission. Let me explain.

While researching the sin of gluttony, I found a helpful explanation in Ligonier's *Tabletalk* magazine: "Commonly Tolerated Sins." Yikes. Dr. Burk

Parsons explains the difference between the sins of omission and the sins of commission for our understanding:

> We dare not ignore any sin even as some sins stand out to us more than others, for every sin is a transgression against God and His law. We often hear about the sins that involve our actions but often ignore the sins that involve our failing to act, to do what we are supposed to do. Westminster Shorter Catechism 14 reminds us that sin is any want of conformity unto the law of God (sins of omission) or any transgression of that law (sins of commission). We have a tendency to overlook our own sins while highlighting the sins of others.
>
> Yet we ought always to strive to hate our sins more than the sins of other Christians who sin differently than we do. May we never overlook our own sins as we pray that God opens our eyes to see those sins that we may be blind to, always remembering that there is more grace in God than sin in us.[36]

Again, I remind you that I can't decide for you if your food behavior is sinful. That's between you and God. But what I can do is confess to you that food was an idol in my life for at least thirty long years and show you a practical way through this battle.

In the same *Tabletalk* edition, I found a short article on gluttony, you know, that tolerated sin no one wants to speak about. Well, it's my privilege to exhort you with some hard truths through my personal experiences. Then you can ask yourself if this is you.

I appreciate the gentle but firm manner in which Dr. Guy M. Richard handles this topic in his article about gluttony.

"Many commonly tolerated sins are coping mechanisms. They are attempts to fill up what is lacking in our lives and are idols of our own making."[37] Does that put a check in your spirit? It sure did for me.

"As John Calvin once said, our hearts really are 'idol factories' that constantly manufacture new gods for us to serve."[38] With a heart transformed, I realized I had exhausted myself creating these gods. How about you? Are you exhausted?

"Food gives us a sense of comfort and a sense of being in control, at least in some way."[39] Admittedly, I would say in a whole lot of ways. I craved that control! Does food control you?

"Gluttony turns to food for comfort, joy, endurance, and contentment rather than to God. It loves the gift more than the Giver."[40] I was stuffing the holes in my soul with food. Where are you finding your contentment and joy?

I appreciate Dr. Richard's biblical emphasis regarding gluttony: "In the Bible it is more narrowly considered as overindulgence in one specific area—namely, eating food."[41] Yep, now we've arrived at the heart of the matter. So, what are we to do?

First, can we admit to ourselves that we have our little hissy fits with the mindset of "She can eat whatever she wants! It's not fair! Why can't I indulge, too?"

My friend, I share this with you in all gentleness and love. We can't compare ourselves to what she can do because God created her uniquely, and she has a different metabolism than you and I. And besides, how do we know she isn't skinny fat (skinny on the outside, fat on the inside) and secret-eating, too?

It's a hard truth if we tolerate the sin of gluttony and remain stuck in it. We can't indulge because often we overindulge. And I don't know about you, but I'm uncomfortable with the idea of overindulgence at His table in the heavenly realms.

Let's look up again. Picture yourself at this heavenly table. Consider again *where we long to be* and our invitation to be seated with Christ in the heavenly realms (Ephesians 2:6). This verse even says that God raised us to take this seat as His table. Hallelujah! Here is your hope, not to mention your invitation. Let's go prepared.

And how do we prepare? Review *where we've been* and *where we are* as we present ourselves to dine at this table in the heavenly realms. It's everything our heart craves when we consider *where we long to be*.

More specifically, we prepare by setting our minds on the provisions and protection of God in how we care for our health. In this Ephesians 2 passage, we see the path that Paul lays out for our journey. Ask yourself the following questions:

"What were (or are) my cravings for my sinful desires? How often and how easily do my thoughts follow these unhealthy cravings?"

"Where have I been? Where am I now?"

"Can I see the way out?" Hint: Look for God's grace and mercy.

"Where and how do I get to where my heart craves and longs to be?" Remember: God raised and seated you with Christ in the heavenly realms. There is a seat for you.

Ah, *heavenly*. This is our focus. This represents our future—the day we experience full body, mind, and spirit healing. This, dear reader, is my focus all day, every day: heaven. I keep my mind fixed on heaven, envisioning Jesus at the head of that table while the rest of us laugh and enjoy nourishment the way God designs. The fellowship sounds amazing.

Keeping this vision of the future in my mind gives me peace, joy, and satisfaction because God now controls my cravings. And He will deliver another good gift to help you here on earth—*the gift of self-control*. You can control your cravings. You can. And when you do, you will experience the greatest victory in your freedom story.

Instead of allowing fleshly cravings to rule your day, I invite you to join me in pursuing the true fruit that satisfies the longings of your heart. Even though I don't eat much fruit, this is the fruit I recommend daily.

But the fruit of the spirit is love, joy, peace, patience, kindness, goodness, faithfulness, gentleness, and *self-control*. Against such things there is no law. Those who belong to Christ Jesus have crucified the sinful nature with its passions and desires. Since we live by the Spirit, let us keep in step with the Spirit. (Galatians 5:22–25, emphasis mine)

Taking control of your cravings becomes a daily mindset mission. Remember daily that God created you for a unique purpose and provides the power and the way to overcome your food and sugar cravings for His excellent plan and glory.

We've spent this entire section leaning on God in the hard work of renewing your mind. You can flip your mindset script with God's help (managing those nagging thoughts and emotions), destroy old patterns of behavior (He is able), leave your failures behind (the past is in your rear-view mirror), and control your fleshly cravings.

Now you know this is hard but very important work. You can accomplish this through your commitment to your spiritual sanctification journey.

Let's move forward into our next section, "Redeeming Your Spirit," and seek God to redeem our spiritual walk for our whole health.

A Note to Your Former Self:

A Note to Your Future Self:

Transform-Action Task:

Section 4: Redeeming Your Spirit

■ ■ ■

Redeem (verb): to free from what distresses or harms: such as;
to free from captivity by payment of ransom;
to extricate from or help to overcome something detrimental;
to release from blame or debt: clear;
to free from the consequences of sin.[42]

Therefore, since we are surrounded by such a great cloud of witnesses,
let us throw off everything that hinders and the sin that so easily
entangles, and *let us run with perseverance* the race marked out for us.
Let us fix our eyes on Jesus, the author and perfecter of our faith,
who *for the joy* set before him endured the cross, scorning its shame,
and sat down at the right hand of the throne of God.
Consider him who endured such opposition from sinful men,
so that you will not grow weary and lose heart.
—Hebrews 12:1–3, emphases mine

Chapter 12

Feasting on God's

Satisfying Word

"I'm positive I wouldn't be sitting around this table with you if your heart had not changed." And she continued with something like, "Your opinions and judgments used to be very off-putting."

Whoa. Interesting.

"I understand what you're saying…" I said, immediately acknowledging and agreeing with her assessment. I praised God for this healing journey and credited the change in my life through my dedication and passion for God's Word.

She finished with, "God has done amazing work in your life." All glory to God! This woman is one of the best supporters of my ministry life. She observed how God's Word changed me.

Do you have people in your life observing your spiritual walk? Take my word for it: they pay attention. Let me be your friend in the manner in which Alice has been a friend to me.

It's time to move into my favorite part of our journey—spiritual health, which is truly the most important aspect of your heart health. Let's begin with the profound questions I have asked myself for years.

Does God really care about our health? Or, more specifically, *Does God call us to care for our complete health—body, mind, and spirit?* And I would even wonder, *Does He have the time to care about little old me? Surely, He has more important matters of concern. Perhaps I'll hide out over here, try to remain unnoticed.* You may know this particular battle in your mind of *avoiding* being seen but *longing* to be seen.

The answers to these questions unfolded before me through the pages of Ephesians, where I discovered God's inviting embrace, beckoning me as He beckons you to partake in His abundant provision. When I feast on His Word first thing daily, that's when the answers come. If you're not in the habit of picking up your Bible, I beg you to put it into practice today. God has something to say to you that is very specific to *you and only you.* Don't miss the message! Yes, you will have to establish this as a daily discipline (include it in your PACT goals), but I promise, before long, it will become your daily delight. I heard my pastor say that for years. Turns out, he was right!

Imagine your joy in the invitation to sit at that table in the heavenly realms. You have an invitation to the Feast of Feasts! Now, feast on God's good smorgasbord in His Word.

Let's head back to Ephesians, a book we rely on heavily for spiritual nourishment. Paul offers important reminders to us as Christ's followers.

> Consequently, you are no longer foreigners and aliens, but fellow citizens with God's people and members of God's household, built on the foundation of the apostles and prophets, with Christ Jesus himself as the chief cornerstone. In him the whole building is joined together and rises to become a holy temple in the Lord. *And in him you too are being built together to become a dwelling in which God lives by his Spirit.* (Ephesians 2:19–22, emphasis mine)

This passage echoes a profound revelation—we are being built together into a *dwelling place* for God by His Spirit. A dwelling place for God. *In us.* Let's explore how God dwells in us.

Contemplating the when and how of God dwelling in us reminds me of the tent of meeting in Moses's time, where God's presence dwelt among His people, guiding them. Then, the temple Solomon built further exemplified this sacred dwelling, where only a select few entered the Holy of Holies, a space sanctified by God's presence. Prophets foretold of a coming Messiah, and when Jesus, fully God and fully man, arrived, He became the tangible embodiment of God dwelling among us. Jesus Incarnate dwelt among us. This is profound!

Reflecting on John 1:14, "The Word became flesh and made his dwelling among us," I envision Jesus walking, teaching, healing, and celebrating life with us. His tangible presence fills my heart with indescribable joy, knowing He understands our struggles intimately.

I marvel at His endurance while fasting for forty days in the wilderness (see Luke 4:1–13), facing immense challenges while Satan lurked nearby. Yet, Jesus, fully divine and fully human, walked alongside us, becoming relatable in our struggles. *Jesus dwelt among us!*

Ephesians 2:22 reiterates: "And in him you too are being built together to become a dwelling in which God lives by his Spirit." This truth astounds me—God's progression from the tent to the temple, to Christ's incarnation, and now dwelling within us by His Spirit. Wow.

Diving deeper into passages from Ephesians, Corinthians, and Romans, Paul's writings resonate deeply in profound ways for us to reflect on. In 1 Corinthians 3:16 (ESV), he exhorts, "Do you not know that you are God's temple and that God's Spirit dwells in you?" Our bodies are sanctified, sacred, and indwelt by the Holy Spirit, urging us to honor God in all we do. This encompasses abstaining from immorality and acknowledging our bodies as temples of God's presence.

First Corinthians 6:19 reinforces this truth: "Your body is a temple of the Holy Spirit who is in you." This reminder urges us to honor God by abstaining from sin while caring for our bodies—shunning gluttony, embracing holistic wellness, and honoring Him in every aspect of life.

Don't forget that, as Paul wrote in Ephesians 2, we are *made alive in Christ*! Paul reminds us again in this passage in Romans:

In the same way, count yourselves dead to sin but alive to God in Christ Jesus. Therefore do not let sin reign in your mortal body so that you obey its evil desires. Do not offer the parts of your body to sin, as instruments of wickedness, but rather offer yourselves to God, as those who have been brought from death to life; and offer the parts of your body to him as instruments of righteousness. For sin shall not be your master because you are not under the law, but under grace. (Romans 6:11–14)

This passage should prompt us to view ourselves as alive to God in Christ Jesus, rejecting sin's dominion over us and offering our bodies as instruments of righteousness. Paul challenges us, showing the steps to *freedom and victory in Christ*—living for God, refusing to let sin reign, and offering ourselves wholly to Him. It is the pursuit of holiness. Is it hard? Yes. Does Paul offer a strong call to action? Again, yes. Place yourself at that table, alive in Christ, and feast on these exhortations.

Contemplating these Scriptures, allow yourself to ponder the immense freedom you have in Christ—freedom from captivity, vitality in your journey, and the calling God places upon each of us. Paul's teachings illuminate our capacity for experiencing abundant life in Christ.

Returning to *dwell*, let's explore its deeper meanings—abiding as a resident, acknowledging God's perpetual presence within us. This realization demands introspection as we wrestle with the implications of God residing within us.

Acknowledging God *dwells* in us, I urge you to honor God in every aspect of your being—body, mind, spirit, emotions, and relationships—for His glory. As your transformative action task, I encourage you to reflect on these verses. Contemplate how you can glorify the God who dwells in you in every dimension of your life.

But How Can Words Satisfy My Hunger?

I'm delighted you asked! Because I wonder—have you tried daily Bible time? Are you soaking in the presence of God through reading Scripture, prayer, and worship? Where is this discipline on your to-do list? Do you find yourself distracted by your daily tasks and chores or by the strong pull of other means of comfort? Like scrolling social media or Netflix bingeing, for example? Don't forget the mindless snacking in front of the TV. Would you believe me if I told you that soaking in dedicated time with God daily has not only flipped the cravings of my life but richly satisfied every longing, every hunger, and every craving in my soul?

I never want to make it sound easier said than done because I don't know your circumstances. But David also testifies in Psalm 40, "God put a new song in my mouth, a hymn of praise. Many will see and fear and put their trust in the Lord."

Well, I have tasted and seen what spiritual health compared to spiritual apathy looks like up close and personal, so I can testify. Remember in my introduction, I referred to myself as a *casual Christian*? Let me explain.

Do you have casual acquaintances in your life? You know, those people you bump into at your local market and will spend thirty minutes catching up on life, kids, and community events? Let's be honest: you enjoy these people and might even say you love them—or at least you love spending time with them. But when you agree to *get together and catch up later...* it never happens. You have great intentions, but your follow-through stinks. Like so many great ideas in your life, reacquainting yourselves slips through the cracks. Again. and yeah, you feel a little guilty, but you get over it fast because you are *so busy*!

That perfectly describes the old me and my casual approach to Jesus. Over years of attending church and women's Bible study groups, I enjoyed bumping into Jesus occasionally. It hurts my heart to admit this to you, but in hindsight, I know the lack of depth in our relationship rested solely with me. I never spent time getting to know Jesus intimately through God's Word. Nor through prayer and a true heart of worship. Here we are, back to the heart of the matter. *The heart*!

For decades, I lived with a dissatisfied heart. I suppose I could make the excuse that I didn't know any better. This is partially true because, recognizing the immense satisfaction found in God's Word, I wish I could instantly change my past and start reading my Bible daily from the time I was able to read. But again, hindsight is always 20/20, right? I'm sharing my hindsight with you as foresight for your future self. Your future health in body, mind, and spirit. And, of course, your heart.

Not only did I lack the spiritual nourishment from feasting on God's Word daily, but if you took a magnifying glass to examine my heart (think about that scene from *How the Grinch Stole Christmas*), you'd see a heart ten sizes too small. Day to day, you'd find me moody but doing my very best to live up to appearances' sake of a woman all put together. Being happy when walking around daily with a broken heart is hard. And let's not forget about the opinions and judgments I shared on social media. Yikes. I believed I was *right,* if you catch my meaning, but I learned from an honest friend how wrong I had been.

I'll never forget the conversation above with dear Alice, a woman from my church. Gathered around a table of women, I don't recall what prompted the conversation, but I'll never forget her words. I've come a long way in this healing journey!

Now, I find satisfaction in feasting on God's Word daily, and it does fill me up. It fills me up to overflowing, creating a passion to pass it along to you and my clients. As much as I want you to lose weight for your quality of life, exhorting women to pick up the Word is my number-one passion. Hearing testimonies of life change fills my heart with joy and excites me to share a remarkable testimony with you.

Meet a client who embraced my coaching advice, delving into the Book of Proverbs and reaping a treasure trove of wisdom and satisfaction. Athena's journey isn't just about her weight-loss success; it's a testament to the immeasurable power of diving deep into God's Word. Don't just take my word for it—take notes from Athena's story, a story of witnessing firsthand the profound impact of embracing God's truth to satisfy every heart craving.

––––––

Athena Dean Holtz—My Journey from Cravings to Contentment

I'm Athena. I'm excited to share my journey, which intertwines deeply with this chapter. God's Word is a satisfying feast, and Christine's invaluable coaching significantly impacted my experience in battling weight loss.

My path wasn't a straight line; it was a winding road tangled with the struggles of emotional eating, cravings, and the deceptive allure they carried. Enter Christine's coaching—a beacon of light that led me through a transformative revelation—the incomparable power in God's Word.

During our coaching sessions, we delved into Proverbs 4:20–27, unlocking a reservoir of wisdom tailor-made for my struggles. Those verses resonated deeply within my soul, guiding me to pay attention to God's words regarding my health, lean into His sayings, and fiercely guard my heart from the clutches of deceit. I discovered life, health, and unwavering stability amid life's tempests in embracing His truth. Read the wisdom found in this proverb:

My son, pay attention to my words; incline your ear to my sayings. Do not lose sight of them; keep them within your heart. For they are life to those who find them, and health to the whole body. Guard your heart with all diligence, for from it flow springs of life. Put away deception from your mouth; keep your lips from perverse speech. Let your eyes look forward; fix your gaze straight ahead. Make a level path for your feet, and all your ways will be sure. Do not swerve to the right or to the left; turn your feet away from evil. (Proverbs 4:20–27 BSB)

I couldn't ignore the parallels—how our cravings, whether for food, substances, or enticing promises, ensnare us in a cycle of deception. They entrap us and weave deceitful webs that capture those around us. It was a powerful realization. But this passage in Proverbs provides a clear path to freedom from our food struggles. I identified eleven crucial truths, my action steps, from this passage:

Pay attention to His words. This initial step involves more than mere reading; it's about active listening. Dive deep into God's Word, not merely scanning but intentionally absorbing every syllable. Listen to His voice speaking through Scripture, allowing His wisdom to resonate deeply within your soul.

Incline our ear to His sayings. It's not just about listening but leaning in, eagerly seeking to grasp the profound meaning behind His teachings. Incline your heart to receive His words, understanding that His sayings hold the keys to transformation and wisdom beyond measure.

Keep them (His words) in sight. Beyond absorbing His words now, imagine His teachings even in the busiest moments, anchoring yourself in His truth as a constant guide through life's twists and turns.

Keep them in your heart. Let His words take residence within you. Internalize them so profoundly that they become the guiding compass in every decision, radiating through your thoughts, actions, and interactions with others. Read them in the first person, out loud!

Guard your heart with all diligence. Protect this sacred dwelling place of His words. Shield your heart from influences that contradict His teachings, nurturing an environment where His truth thrives, and deceit finds no foothold.

Put away deception. This step involves a deliberate effort to cast away falsehood and deception. Embrace honesty and authenticity in every aspect of life, aligning your thoughts and words with God's truth, even when it hurts to stand up for the Truth.

Keep your lips from perverse speech. Let the purity of His words shape your speech. Guard your tongue against deceit and crookedness, allowing only words that reflect His truth and grace to flow from your lips.

Look and gaze forward, straight ahead. Fix your gaze on the path illuminated by His truth. Keep your focus on the journey ahead, guided by His teachings, avoiding distractions that veer you off course.

Make a level path forward. Smooth out the rough patches in your journey. Create an environment conducive to growth, ensuring that every step parallels His truth, paving the way for a purposeful walk in faith.

Do not swerve right or left. Remain steadfast on the course set by His Word. Refrain from veering off into distractions or temptations that deviate from His truth, remaining resolute in your commitment to follow His guidance.

Turn your feet away from evil. Take deliberate steps away from anything contrary to His teachings. Choose righteousness over evil, allowing His Word to guide your actions and lead you away from paths that diverge from His truth.

Reflecting upon this transformative journey taught me a fundamental truth: elevating anything above God binds us in chains. My journey became about relinquishing these idols, inviting God's Spirit to flood every void within me, guiding me along a path illuminated by His timeless truths and liberating grace. Embracing the action steps, I give God all the glory for His Word's benefits over my whole health journey. Perks such as:

Life to those who find them.
Health to your whole body.

Springs of life flowing.
All your ways will be sure.

Sharing my story isn't merely about laying bare my struggles; it's about embracing the whispers of God's loving call to transformation and finding profound healing through the pages of His Word.

So, here's the heart of the matter: What have you concealed in your life that God has tenderly brought into the light? How did you respond when faced with His beckoning toward transformation?

Christine's coaching was pivotal in this expedition, steering me toward a feast on God's Word—an adventure filled with solace, healing, and an unmatched sense of freedom in embracing His eternal truths. I pray you will experience this freedom as you dine on God's satisfying Word through your health and healing journey.

———

I'm extremely proud of Athena's weight-loss victory. She's lost over forty pounds and is maintaining a healthy weight. Athena is not alone in discovering the true source of nourishment for physical, emotional, and spiritual health. It's only when we embrace this most important aspect of our whole being that transformation begins to take hold in our hearts. Now, you may be wondering how you can do the same.

From Casual to Committed

Around 2011, I recall seeing tons of bumper stickers on cars during a movement from a large local church called the *2WordStory*. This happened during my casual Christian years. Seeing the stickers everywhere piqued my curiosity, so I did a little research to understand. A *2WordStory* is one word with a double meaning—from something negative to a positive. The idea invited you to testify with just one word about how Jesus changed your life. I remember trying to come up with a word during this season of my life. Reflecting on that time, I experienced exhaustion every day. Would Jesus move me from exhaustion to exhaustion? I don't think so. I never came up with my own *2WordStory* when the movement was popular, but that catchy phrase never left my thoughts for some reason.

It's so apparent to me now why I couldn't choose a word as a sporadic church attender and, more importantly, someone who rarely picked up the word of God. My heritage of faith provided head knowledge of God's Word but sorely lacked heart knowledge. And I'll repeat it: this holistic health and wellness journey is all about the heart, and that requires … action!

Sporadically, I would attend Bible study at my friend Tammy's house. My rebellious heart chuckled to itself when the Bible study teacher leaned toward the camera and said, "I want you to pray to God to start waking you up at 5:00 a.m. so that you can begin your day with Him."

"Lady, there is no way I am praying to God to wake me up early every day! I'm exhausted." There's my word again—*exhausted*!

I barely got my lessons done to prep for the study group. I'm terribly guilty of cramming my homework and only checking it off my to-do list for appearance's sake. Can you relate?

Do you believe God has a sense of humor? That He is good and fun? Let me tell you something funny. Very early in my healing journey (and after I came home with that CPAP machine), I began waking up around 5:00 a.m. every morning without an alarm. That woman's exhortation became my reality! I'm still chuckling.

I began picking up my Bible in those early morning hours for the first time, and I haven't put it down since! Beginning my day in the quiet and stillness of my home while listening to God's still, small voice flipped my life upside down in ways I had never imagined. Has this happened to you, too? Or will you allow this to happen to you?

I'm not a breakfast eater, but this is all the nourishment I need to begin each day. God's Word, this feast, satisfies every longing, craving, and hole in my soul. You can quickly patch up those holes by applying (acting upon) the truths and promises gifted to us through God's Holy Word.

And now I have my *2WordStory*! Reflecting on my chronic health issues and constant companion of exhaustion and attempting to do all the right things for my health that repeatedly failed … I lived *overwhelmed*. *Overwhelmed* by every aspect of my life—physically, emotionally, and spiritually.

But God. I love those two words! God, He's the source of my new *overwhelmed* life! My heart is overwhelmed by all His provision, providence, and plan for a healthy life. God gives good gifts to *overwhelm* the soul. Gifts like:

- Whole foods to heal our whole health.
- Fruits of the spirit—my passion for joy while also enjoying love, peace, patience, kindness, goodness, faithfulness, gentleness, and self-control. (See Galatians 5)
- His written Word. (Consider that much of the world cannot access a Bible.)
- The body of Christ—for fellowship and community. (I'm glad you're here.)

I could go on, but you get the idea. Take time to jot down how God is *overwhelming* your life. If you don't feel overwhelmed by His goodness, what's your next step to get there?

Friend, if you are feeling broken-hearted, exhausted, or all the things we often think about our poor health, please take my advice. If you take nothing else from this book, I pray you take the advice to satisfy your hunger with God's Word daily. May this journey deepen your understanding of God's invitation to feast on His Word and cultivate a holistic connection between body, mind, and spirit for His ultimate glory. "You show up, God shows off!"

A Note to Your Former Self:

A Note to Your Future Self:

Transform-Action Task:

CHAPTER 13

SURRENDERING STRONGHOLDS AND SHATTERING THE SUGAR SHACKLES

■ ■ ■

The weight of my circumstances for thirty years became too much to bear. I craved the sound of freedom. Imagine hearing the sounds of chains rattling to chains breaking—the only way to hear this freedom song is through the eyes of your heart. Your heart transformation. With heartfelt actions of surrender. Not just once, but daily. Over and over and over again. It's an important strategy, so don't skim this chapter.

First, let's frame this entire chapter with this question: "*Is sugar a stronghold in my life?*" Not just sugar, let's include junk food and unhealthy behavior toward food (like secret eating and overindulgence). Please keep in mind that these behaviors, also including gluttony and carelessness, lead to a plethora of chronic and deadly diseases, like obesity, heart disease, type 2 diabetes, and more.

Are you chained down by the weight of your daily food choices? Here is hope. Jesus came to set us free. He invites us to approach His throne with confidence to receive this freedom. This journey to spiritual health requires acts of surrender. It will require a lengthy process and many bandages to bind up the old wounds that have kept you chained to unhealthy food behavior. I call the weight of these chains the *sugar shackles*.

Bunker down. I'm about to call you to live uncomfortably. Fortunately, God's Word provides a plan to comfort your heart.

Don't forget the questions: "*Is sugar a stronghold in my life? Is junk food?*" Remember, when I talk about sugar, I'm not just talking about the sweet stuff. I'm also talking about the highly refined carbohydrates prevalent in our Western diet.

Recall that 60 to 65 percent of our standard American diet is carbohydrates, which break down immediately into sugar during digestion. So, sugar, highly refined carbohydrates, and a diet high in carbohydrates are damaging and destroying our metabolic health, leading to obesity. Some of us have morbid obesity, some of us are just a little bit overweight, and we can't figure out how counting calories and all the things are not working for us. So, this is faith-based encouragement (refer to the section "Restoring Your Body" for the metabolic lessons).

At some point in my Bible, I recorded a fantastic roadmap in Psalm 32. Grab your journal or write in the margins to remember this forever. King David understood the necessary steps to a true heart transformation. He wrote a step-by-step plan for approaching the throne confidently, approaching Jesus confidently, and receiving clarity from Him on what He is calling us to surrender. The transformation steps written in my margin include *promises, admission, confession, thanksgiving, wisdom,* and *praise.*

The Promises of God

David wrote:

> Blessed is he whose transgressions are forgiven, whose sins are covered. Blessed is the man whose sin the Lord does not count against him and in whose spirit is no deceit." (Psalm 32:1–2)

In these first two verses of Psalm 32, David shared the promise of God as a reminder of His goodness. God is always good, even when He calls us to step up and step out into the most uncomfortable unknown.

God is calling you to the most important matters of your heart while reminding you of His love. He knows we struggle and our strongholds. But look at God's goodness. He forgives our sins and can still bless us in this process and journey. Hallelujah!

We identified those sins while working through Susanna Wesley's quote in chapter 8, "Flipping the Mindset Script." Well, those sins are covered if you have accepted God's plan of salvation in your heart. However, it's not enough to remain here. As Christ's followers, we must follow His heart for His plan and good purpose in our lives, and we have much more work to do. And I get it; it's hard to admit. Thinking back to the depravity in my heart, it hurts! But since you've begun the work to handle your emotions, examine your thoughts (and your heart), and have been bold to ask for motivation, you're set up to move into these next steps with courage and action.

Admission—Depart from Apathy

Let's move on to verses three and four. We see David show up authentically and vulnerably, encouraging us to do the same:

When I kept silent, my bones wasted away through my groaning all day long. For day and night your hand was heavy upon me; my strength was sapped as in the heat of summer. (Psalm 32:3–4)

We've gone from the promise to the admission. David admitted to the Lord the depravity deep in his soul, down to his bones. Reflecting on my journey, I find it interesting how difficult it was to admit these heavy burdens that kept me in chains. Not only to myself; I never shared the depths of my despair with anyone. Not even God. Does that sound like you? Do you wake up daily to feel such a heaviness in your spirit? It's challenging to identify. And, of course, I knew my physical health was way out of control, but I didn't get to the point where I was able to admit it truthfully first to myself, then to God.

And admitting it out loud to people in our lives...well, the idea is dreadful. But speaking with women I coach, they do admit things about their health journey. It's been fascinating because we often don't want to admit this pain, do we? However, I remind you of one primary purpose for writing this book for you. You must show up for yourself and, in return, allow God to show off all He did for you. I have an example of an admission story for you.

I'd love to introduce you to Christina and her authentic and vulnerable story. She's admitting much to admonish you to do the same. Christina was among the first to come to me in 2017 as she recognized my drastic weight loss—she's one of the first I sat with over coffee. At the time, I didn't realize it was coaching. Still, because she was the first person to act on my encouragement to quit sugar and found freedom in Christ when she chose well, I recognize now that coaching is what God called me to do in this new and exciting season of life.

Christina has no hesitation in admitting that she's a work-in-process, so we will pick up her story with where she is today.

———

Christina England—Surrendering the Stronghold

I remember the day my dear friend looked me straight in the eye with the gentlest conviction I've ever received. She said, "It's one thing to understand how to eat healthy, but it's something entirely different to understand how God changes our hearts through it. Christina, what is God teaching you through your health and wellness journey?"

What is He teaching me, aside from "eat this, don't eat that?"

It has always made sense to me that God cares about our wellness. Our bodies are His temple. But when Christine encouraged me to go deeper with God in this pursuit, my eyes opened beyond my wildest imagination. She connected the physical with the spiritual in a way I had never considered. You see, I am a recovering emotional eater and full-fledged food addict. For most of my life, I've run to food for comfort on many levels. In good times and bad, food was ever faithful.

"*Or was it?*" That ever-faithful friend brought me to depression, anxiety, super morbid obesity, and more. *What kind of friend does that?*

Staying connected with Christine, her coaching and encouragement helped me discover where my negative relationship with food began. Christine challenged me to ask hard questions and dared me to be brutally honest with myself.

Why did I turn to food as my emotional bandage? What caused this unhealthy attachment? Even more important, was I willing to allow God to fill that void instead of food?

It truly is mind-boggling to me that I never realized it before then, but Christine asked the right questions and helped me understand my deeply rooted trauma in a whole new light. Food became my nemesis when I was eight years old. That was a long time ago! So now what? How do I use that information to heal this unhealthy relationship? How do I reconcile years and years of bad choices to turn my life around? Through a steadfast pursuit of a deeper relationship with Jesus. I know that sounds overly simplistic, but it isn't. The answer *is* that easy; living it out is not as easy.

Christine always says, "This will be one of the hardest things you will ever do." She is 100 percent correct. While I am far from my goal physically, emotionally, or spiritually, I know I am well on my way. I've grown emotionally and spiritually. I read my Bible and pray every day without fail. It's the first thing I do in the morning. I look forward to that time with Jesus more than anything. He is my strength, my portion, my song.

Physically, I no longer need a cane to walk; I have lost a substantial amount of weight and continue to get stronger. This journey reaches highs; this journey skims some lows. The road hasn't been steady or consistent. I've made mistakes, but I'm confident the battle is already won. I know I will overcome because I'm in the Word every day. Every day, I wake up and pray that I will choose Jesus over food. Every day, I pray that He sanctifies me more to His likeness and grants complete victory over this battle. One day, I know He will.

I am forever grateful to Christine for her friendship, courage to step out of her comfort zone, and the wisdom she willingly shares. And for her coaching and caring heart that exhorts me to live comfortably while being uncomfortable for the glory of God.

———

Proud is an understatement when I consider Christina's journey. I remember the days of her walking the aisle in our church with her cane. I celebrate with her the fact that she no longer needs that aid. Christina gets to testify how God's good smorgasbord of food heals! Be sure to visit the Resources page for a link to the photo scrapbook for a before and after of each success story.

Acknowledging and admitting the strongholds in her life that were impacting her health set her on a path for Jesus to set her free from the heavy chains—those emotional bandages—and put her on a path to a pain-free life in body, mind, heart, and spirit!

Another story for God's glory. Woohoo!

My friend, are you ready to admit that God has more in store for you? This Sugar*Freed* movement isn't just for you and me—it's for those "who told so and so, who told so and so ... and so on!" There are so many opportunities to share with others who are weighed down by the *sugar shackles*.

Christina's story should inspire you—it's so exciting, right? Of course, it is! Can you admit this as an opportunity for your God-given purpose? Great. We've got a little work to do at the foot of the cross now. Let's head into the next expression of confession from David's psalm.

Confession—Take It to the Cross

David laid out the *promise* of God—the point of *admission* that leads us to *confession*:

> Then I acknowledged my sin to you and did not cover up my iniquity. I said, 'I will confess my transgressions to the Lord'—and you forgave the guilt of my sin. (Psalm 32:5)

Right to the heart of the matter!

You are reading this part because you believe there is a stronghold regarding your health. You may not call it a stronghold, so consider this question. What blocks you from God's calling in your health? Will you identify the cycle that keeps you stuck? What's the root of your food behavior? Spend some time here.

Is there something you need to confess in your life right now? Recall the explanation of "What is a sin?" from Susanna Wesley. It's hard, it's scary, it's difficult, it's vulnerable, it's authentic—but it's where you need to be. It leads to freedom, so trust me and trust God's Word. David is guiding you on your health and wellness journey; you must examine the strongholds, admit them, and confess them before God. What do you turn to when you are dealing with a strong emotion? And it can be anywhere on the feelings wheel spectrum, from despair to delight! Feeling excluded leads to secret eating. Feeling excited leads to overstuffing at celebrations. I think you get the idea.

But don't forget about the *promise* of God that David laid out right at the beginning of this psalm. David said, "And you forgave the guilt of my sin." Guilt. Ugh. That's one of our heaviest chains. Hop back to chapter 10, "Leaving Failures Behind," if you need a reminder to leave that guilt and shame behind!

God forgives the guilt of our sins. He does not want us to carry this extra weight, these extra heavy burdens on our hearts. Even Jesus urges us to:

Come to me, all you who are weary and burdened, and I will give you rest. Take my yoke upon you and learn from me, for I am gentle and humble in heart, and you will find rest for your souls. For my yoke is easy and my burden is light. (Matthew 11:28–30)

What a relief. I would suggest, "Run, run to Him. *Confess* the strongholds holding you down." Once you've done that, we can move forward.

Thanksgiving—From Trouble to a Thankful Heart

What happens when we have a breakthrough? How does your heart feel now? Or how about that weight on your shoulders? Is it gone? Yes? I trust you will feel grateful. Thankful! You've confessed, and God has forgiven you. Hallelujah!

David shared words of thanksgiving for you to emulate:

Therefore let everyone who is godly pray to you while you may be found; surely when the mighty waters rise, they will not reach him. You are my hiding place; you will protect me from trouble and surround me with songs of deliverance." (Psalm 32:6–7)

It sure sounds like a freedom song of *thanksgiving* to me. Deliverance. Woo! Thanksgiving because of what the Lord did for David; He provided David a way out. The songs of deliverance—that's what we're pursuing today and every day into our future of freedom. We're pursuing deliverance from our health struggles. We're pursuing the freedom God offers us over our well-being: body, mind, and spirit. Is your heart overflowing with *thanksgiving* today?

When we admit, confess, and see the Lord working, we regain control of our health and wellness. Don't you feel such relief? Such a release of those heavy chains? God's promises always ring true. And we need to *give thanks* to God for that, right? Where do we go from here? Let's seek *wisdom* in His Word. It's time to act on David's next part of the plan in Psalm 32.

Wisdom—Found in God's Word

David continues his instruction with *wisdom* gleaned from the Lord:

I will instruct you and teach you in the way you should go; I will counsel you and watch over you. Do not be like the horse or the mule, which have no understanding but must be controlled by bit and bridle or they will not come to you. Many are the woes of the wicked, but the Lord's unfailing love surrounds the man whose trust is in him. (Psalm 32:9–10)

Trust is in Him. Do you trust God for your whole health? Do you trust God in your journey? I wrote *wisdom* next to these three verses.

God is with you on this journey, instructing you and guiding you. If you follow Christ, the Holy Spirit will guide and nudge you. He nudged you to do something about your health, which is why you picked up this book.

I love hearing your stories, so don't hesitate to share whatever wisdom God puts in your heart to help others. People need to listen to the life-giving knowledge you've gained in your health. Remember my purpose? For the healing wisdom to share … and so on and so on! Because I know in my journey as I began healing, I woke up many days and said, "Wow, I can't believe this. God's Word is full of exhortation for me on how I care for my body, mind, spirit, and heart." And I missed it for all those years. But I discovered *wisdom* in His Word. So, my friend, if you are reading this and not reading His Word, I invite you to begin picking up your Bible. Grab it and flip to Psalm 32 with me. I'll wait!

I encourage you to instill this practice daily because that's where you will be nourished and find satisfaction and support—and *wisdom*. How will your knowledge grow if you're not reading these words? I'm just here as a woman blessed by the goodness of God, listening and responding to what He was putting on my heart through the nudging of the Holy Spirit.

"What's my next step, Lord? What's my next step? Just continue to teach me. Help me heal. Help me heal physically. Help me heal emotionally. Help me heal spiritually. Heal my heart, Lord!"

There is wisdom. Right there in your Bible. I can pass on what I know about this lifestyle as a coach. I can guide you, but the wisdom you need genuinely comes from God Himself.

All right, we've gone from *promise* to *admission* to *confession* to *thanksgiving* to *wisdom* from God's Word. "Taste and see that the Lord is good; blessed is the man who takes refuge in him" (Psalm 34:8).

Trust me. If you don't trust me in anything else through this book journey, trust me in gleaning your wisdom daily from Scripture. It will change your life (just like it changed mine). Reading my Bible has filled my heart with greater joy and delivered me to freedom. I can't help but rejoice in songs of praise.

Praise—Pour It Out!

David wrapped up this psalm with a call to *praise* and worship:

> Rejoice in the Lord and be glad, you righteous; sing all you who are upright in heart. (Psalm 32:11)

You know I'm all about the joy, right? I love the fruit of the spirit joy.

Joy changed my life. Joy transformed my heart. You know by now that that true transformation in *The* Sugar*Freed Method* is the heart transformation. It's the very foundation of this journey that we're on, my friend. And once we see it, we can't unsee it.

Getting down to the nitty-gritty heart of the matter should prompt you to quiet your heart today and spend time in Psalm 32—time in your journal writing about God's *promises*, your *admission*, your *confession*, and your song of *thanksgiving*. Lean on the Lord for greater *wisdom* in caring for your body, mind, heart, and spirit. Ask the Lord for a new level of motivation today.

Ask God to guide you from the desert place into those songs of deliverance. I will never return to that desert place despite God taking me through different seasons of life since I've regained my health. I've had severe and complicated struggles. Suffering I never anticipated. Moments in my life that hurt my heart to the core. These situations come in cycles and are present in my life as I write.

Sharing with my therapist the other day, she inquired, "How are you processing this?" I sighed and replied, "Well, I didn't process it with food!" Whenever that truth pops into my mind, I remind myself of God's great plan to help us live free! And I never take for granted the miracle of being set free from decades of sugar and food addiction.

But remember, I say I'm a recovering sugar and food addict. Because when the days do get hard, it is a battle, but an altogether worthy battle— one worth fighting. It's a battle I long for you to stop losing, too. Today is the day to begin declaring your victory. Will you fight for it?

Losing weight will be a wonderful gift, and it comes from seeking the Lord for guidance. For your step-by-step guide, you can repeatedly return to Psalm 32: *Promises, Admission, Confession, Thanksgiving, Wisdom, Praise*.

When my client, Sara (whom you met in chapter 7), heard my lesson on Psalm 32, she chimed in, "God is so sweet to start the psalm with the sure promise of His forgiveness." Amen to that, Sara.

This important heart work will help you step up and step out into God's calling on your life while healing your body, mind, and spirit. God will show off in your healing story. Are you ready? This leads me to encourage you to show up without fear.

A Note to Your Former Self:

A Note to Your Future Self:

Transform-Action Task:

CHAPTER 14

CONQUERING FEAR

■ ■ ■

If you force me to choose one spiritual battle that impacted my life the most throughout my weight-loss journey—the answer is *fear*. Clinically, it's known as anxiety. I feel compelled to share this part of the journey with you because as you heal spiritually, I wholeheartedly believe that God will call you to share your story for His glory. Don't be afraid. It's one of the most satisfying aspects of this journey. Trust me! People need to hear this message on repeat.

As I contemplate my almost fifty years before healing, I realize fear left me with many battle scars—scars I don't enjoy looking at but are essential to examine. As the scars fade, my resolve develops, protecting me from the wounds of fear.

Writing this book, I realized several topics overlapped with emotional and spiritual healing. I decided to discuss *fear* in this section. I'll explain why I put it here about my spiritual healing, but first, I want to define *fear*.

Fear noun:

1a: an unpleasant, often strong emotion caused by anticipation or awareness of danger
b: **(1):** an instance of this emotion
(2): a state marked by this emotion
2: anxious concern: solicitude
3: profound reverence and awe especially toward God
4: reason for alarm: danger

Fear verb: transitive verb

1: to be afraid of: expect with alarm *fear* the worst
2: to have a reverential awe of *fear* of God
3: *archaic*: frighten
4: *archaic*: to feel fear in (oneself)[43]

Pay particular attention to the definitions above. I see explanations for our carnal and innate human response, plus descriptions of how we respond to God. My understanding of fear has deepened in both regards. I'm a little afraid (see what I did there?) to pour out my heart on this topic, so I trust these words will flow through the Holy Spirit.

I lived my life in fear. The shame of my physical appearance often made me hide away. Walking into a crowded room often paralyzed me, so I found it easier to avoid. As a result, I lived my life in a comfortable level of isolation. Sure, my family and close friends were not a threat, but I never engaged on a deeper level with the place God calls us all to be. Right under my nose, I had an entire body of believers for fellowship, encouragement, uplifting, and accountability. Why was I so hesitant to engage?

I was afraid to walk into the room. First, what if I didn't know anyone? Or worse yet, what if someone I do know doesn't have a seat at her table? Then, I would have to walk around awkwardly until I could find a seat.

And if those feelings aren't bad enough, what if I'm the fattest girl in the room? Truthfully, my thoughts always went there. I'm sorry to say, but they did. Always. Do you share those thoughts?

Even before I entered the door, I knew deep down that I would be the fattest, most shameful girl in the room. As an obese woman, I never thought there was a seat for me at any table. That was my thinking—is this messed up, or can you relate?

Wait, there's more. As I walked into the room, I experienced a deep sense of dread if the event centered around food. Indeed, I imagined all judging eyes were upon me as I moved the fork up and down. "Why is she eating that?"

You get the idea. I was frightened to deal with the fear of walking into a room. I bet there is a phobia word to describe this. My level of this type of fear was not as debilitating as agoraphobia because I never struggled to leave the house to shop and run errands. It seems I experienced social anxiety based on my appearance and inability to process my emotions. So, I stayed home. I stayed home from Christmas parties, I stayed home from women's ministry events, and I stayed home from high school and college reunions. I stayed home from meetings, even those God prompted me to attend. Sometimes, friends or family could drag me away into this or that type of event, but every time, my body, mind, and spirit filled with dread. Can you relate? Rushing blood, racing heart, averting eyes. Their eyes on me left me wondering how to hide my obese self.

Besides the fear of walking into a room, my insecurities manifested into an intense fear of speaking. Why would anyone be interested in hearing what I have to say?

If you don't understand this yet, be prepared: people treat me much differently now that I am thinner than they did when I was fat. My heart breaks as I process this reality and relive these emotions. I'm sorry to dump this on you. I only hope to encourage us all to be kinder and better humans.

My soul holds no bitterness towards the society which instilled this fear of speaking. I forgive my fellow humans for treating me this way because now I have a lot to say, and I'll never stop talking. Think of it as payback (ha). Sorry, not sorry. I've been catching up on speaking the truth for all the years I was silent.

Before I conquer fear, I need to share a few more fears I battled to unburden them from my soul.

Fear of failure. Fear of losing control. Fear of ridicule. Fear of harm to my children. Fear of losing everything (job, financial stability). Fear of my loved ones facing painful health diagnoses. And, of course, you remember my anxiety over my health diagnoses and challenges. Death at an early age was my motivating fear in this journey. Missing out on my children's adult journeys and never meeting my future grandchildren shook me to the core.

Fear of writing this book. So much fear. How could I, a nobody previously paralyzed by fear, write a book for the world to read? Or not read? Fear of rejection and failure loomed large over the very early stages of this prompting God put on my heart. Really, God? A book? I'll share more about how this book came to be as we explore this chapter.

I've realized several things about my human fear through this raging battle.

Fear is a liar. Fear holds us back. Fear paralyzes. Fear prevents us from living an abundant life. Fear makes us ineffective in our calling. Fear is a spirit. Check out this reminder from Paul to Timothy:

> For God gave us a spirit not of fear but of power and love and self-control. (2 Timothy 1:7 ESV)

Where, my friends, do you think this spirit of fear comes from? It certainly doesn't come from our loving Father. Our Father loves us and longs for us to live free from fear. His heart for us shines through in this verse. By the way, I claim this as my banner verse in my battle to conquer fear. Shortly after I reached my weight-loss goals, the Lord put this verse in my path, and He has been proving Himself true to His promise every day since. It's almost like He whispered, "Alrighty, step one accomplished—you've healed physically. I'll equip you with the flame you need in your next battle." Time to confront fear face-to-face.

Besides knowing that the spirit of fear is not from the Lord, look at what He does give you: Power. Love. And *self-control*. Remember, this was our big lesson from chapter 11, "Controlling Cravings"?

Self-control is essential. I remind you that it impacts your spiritual health. We know that losing weight and regaining our health takes considerable self-control. And look where self-control comes from—it comes from the Lord.

The definition of self-control is restraint exercised over one's impulses, emotions, or desires.[44]

Have you feared failure in regaining your health? Trust this truth from my experience. As I diligently committed to eating low-carb daily for my health, I gained victory and experienced self-control for the first time. Remember, ditching sugar reduces sugar cravings, and your mindset begins to set you up for success with self-control. When I received this spirit of self-control, I gained victory over food addiction and fear.

The gift of the spirit of self-control is available for you right now. Spend time writing 2 Timothy 1:7 on a notecard and carry it everywhere. Keep it close to your heart when food temptations surround you.

The Lord continued to repeat this verse in my life as I launched out on this healing journey. It was the key verse at my home church's women's ministry event. Yes, friends. With trembling fingers, I registered for this event. Challenging my fears of being seen and unseen, I stepped into that conference, a room full of Jesus girls, every single one of them seen by me and, more importantly, in the eyes of Jesus. This moment in my journey marked a huge milestone.

Until God's power, love, and self-control enveloped me in the depths of my soul, fear trapped me like a gateway drug. It constantly beckoned to a path of disobedience. It kept me from speaking and sharing the good news of the gospel I grew up learning. My unhealthy soul squandered many years while I walked in disobedience. In the New International Version of the verse above, *timid* is used instead of fear. The Greek word in the original text is *deilia,* which translates to timidity, fearfulness, and cowardice. For almost fifty years of my life, I lived timidly. Not something I'm proud to share, but oh, the lessons I have gleaned from my past mistakes through this joyful journey with Jesus prompt me to testify every day.

If your heart races right now, and you think, "I can't battle fear; it's too hard," let me share how I'm finding victory over this paralyzing risk factor in our lives.

As I've shared through my emotional and heart healing, feeling healthy exposed my teachable spirit. I dabbled in sharing my weight-loss story with a close audience on my Facebook page. When I reached my goal in early 2018, my husband and kids strongly encouraged me to share my story with a broader audience.

My Generation Z daughter (a founding member of the generation raised with a solid connection to digital society) constantly harassed me, saying, "Mom, you should start a YouTube channel. You could help so many people."

My Generation X-self replied, "Kaitlin. I am not putting my awkward self on camera for the entire world to see." What I didn't say out loud would shine a light on my fear of mistakes and flaws. Not to mention the sheer horror of being that vulnerable. On YouTube. At the time, I said, "No, thank you."

Well, my daughter was forward thinking in her ideas. YouTube is a fantastic platform for reaching an audience of non-readers. You may like to read, but I also invite you to catch me on YouTube. Honestly, hitting upload on each video quickens my heart with a teeny dose of fear each time, but my heart rate returns to normal quickly now.

Back to the story. I began the battle against fear through God's gift of power, love, and self-control. The event sparked a flame. Soon, I would see evidence of how God was fanning the flame that Paul wrote to Timothy about in the previous verse: "For this reason I remind you to fan into flame the gift of God, which is in you from the laying on of my hands" (2 Timothy 1:6 ESV).

Dynamic speakers repeatedly shared the powerful message from Paul to Timothy during our event. I walked away from that event with an overwhelming sense that God was calling me into obedience. Listen in. Is He calling you to step out in obedience to share your health journey?

Historically, fear stopped me in my tracks despite the constant yearlong nudging of the Holy Spirit to stop wasting my life. I received a specific nudge around this time: stop relying on my powers and the comforts of this world. Stop counting on the financial security of my corporate job. Stop living *normal*, if that makes sense. It's time to step up and step out. I walked out of that building with a book of matches and a fire in my belly to share this good news with you. I wrote in the side margin of my Bible, *holy calling*. No fear. No shame.

I find so much comfort in this second book of Timothy. Like Timothy, I grew up with a godly heritage. And like Timothy, my knees were knocking when God came calling me to act on my story.

These two verses in 2 Timothy empower and equip us to strive to conquer fear constantly. It's a good thing, too, because I would have to lean hard into these lessons to defeat fear.

Good Health Sets You Up for Hard Things—Be Fearless!

Still riding on the flame from the inspiring event, God dropped something in my lap just a few weeks later. I received a random direct message on Twitter from a stranger. Now, I don't typically even open messages from strangers, but I could see the first words of this message.

He messaged, "I wasn't sure why I followed you at first glance at your Twitter bio. I'm not a Christian; I'm a dog (not cat) person and didn't even know what LCHF (low-carb, high-fat) stood for. But something prompted me to look at your Twitter timeline. Low-carb is changing my life."

He shared a bit of his journey and ended his message with this: "So thank you for being there. I joined *DietDoctor.com* based on your pinned tweet and think it will be helpful."

We exchanged a few messages about no sugar and no grains, and then he said, "When you build your website—and you will if that's what you desire—I can at least point you in the right direction because that's what I do."

And that, my friends, is how my story ended up being in your hands today.

I share this story for two reasons. First, it's amazing that God would use a random stranger to face my fear of sharing my story. Second, I followed through on facing this fear, and you can, too.

Finally, I think it's of utmost importance to share that God will equip you to face down fear in ways you might never expect. This spiritual healing is vital for when the storms of life hit.

I celebrated many victories in my new way of living Sugar*Freed*, but six months into my new lifestyle, my son was in a catastrophic car crash. Our family life was about to get extremely difficult as we faced trial after trial of trying first to find a proper diagnosis for his closed head injury and seeking adequate care. It's been a long, hard road.

We are still navigating this trial, and I'll share more in a future book about facing this dreadful season with joy while staring down fear. In this season, because I have conquered fear, I've been able to carry joy and sorrow in the same hand while God is holding us all up in His strong and mighty hand. I credit my ability to face these trials because of this spiritual journey of healing. I shudder as I picture myself huddled in a heap on the floor if God had not redeemed my spiritual walk through His perfect plan for my health.

Best of all. Despite a long, horrendous season of sorrow, I maintained my health and wellness in body, mind, and spirit. My former self would have quickly eaten my feelings to another massive weight gain.

Friend, God can and will equip you in the same way. I realize now how important this part of my healing has been in holding my family together during this tumultuous time. Remember, He has created us uniquely as physical, emotional, and spiritual beings—tightly knit together in wholeness for His glory. Honestly, I consider spiritual healing the most essential part of this journey. Lean in.

Remember, part of my *why* is to be there for my family. My son needs me, and my husband needs me to manage all the details of this for our family. I don't even have to guess who needs you to live your healthiest life—there are certainly people in your life who need you to be the best version of yourself. Especially when the storms hit and fear threatens to wipe you out. Trust this truth: *God did not give you a spirit of fear.*

The battle over fear is by no means completely overcome on earth. In fact, with our innate human nature, victory over our carnal sense of fear will have to wait until we dance in heaven.

I continually resolve to strengthen my desire to be more than a conqueror over fear. And I'm sharing these lessons with you so you will *step up and out without fear.* Walking in the promise that God gives you a spirit of love, power, and self-control—not fear—is essential to living Sugar*Freed.* Why? As you transform your health—in body, mind, and spirit—He will use your victory story for His glory.

Let's not forget God's promise of the spirit of self-control. This gift is vital to living a Sugar*Freed* lifestyle! Grab hold of this gift, and don't let go. As I promised regarding healing your body, the low-carb lifestyle enhances the spirit of self-control.

Tips to Quiet the Fear

Perhaps you're wondering what overcoming fear and anxiety in your health and wellness journey looks like. And perhaps you are unaware of the detriment that fear, anxiety, and worry have on your whole health. Stress manifests in many ways in your body, so you must be ready with your battle plan to defeat fear and anxiety.

Maybe you do not know that anxiety not only hurts your emotional health but can impact your physical health, preventing you from achieving a healthy weight. Also, does God want us to walk through our spiritual life with worry and anxiety running our days? Anxiety is out to sabotage your weight-loss goals. Let's stop it in its tracks now.

You can manage (and yes, even defeat) this stress when you implement these five biblical practices to quiet anxiety. Engaging this enemy of your health is a worthy endeavor to protect and enhance your weight-loss efforts.

1. **Trust God.** Remember that God is in control and has a plan for your life. God is sovereign over every circumstance in your life. Your health, family, finances, and culture we live in. God has ordained your days.

   During my season of trial, God increased my trust, an important gift that helped me manage my anxiety on the days I thought I would drown. This is what I learned: *Trust God's plan. The outcome is in His hands.* "Blessed is the man who makes the LORD his trust, who does not look to the proud, to those who turn aside to false gods" (Psalm 40:4).

2. **Pray.** Bring your worries and fears before God and ask for His peace. Peace is the antidote to an anxious life. Despite my trial ending badly, God's peace reigned in my heart and kept me from backsliding into self-sabotaging food behavior. I'm grateful for this peace and the fact that I've maintained my healthy lifestyle. Without this peace, I believe I easily could have been morbidly obese again.

   Every day, I pray for peace (and all the fruits of the Spirit)—increase them all, Lord! Pray this with me: "But the fruit of the Spirit is love, joy, peace, patience, kindness, goodness, faithfulness, gentleness, and self-control. Against such things there is no law" (Galatians 5:22–23).

3. **Read the Bible.** If you only get one takeaway from reading this book, I pray this is it. If you aren't in the habit of reading your Bible daily, I would like to remind you that I picked up my Bible every day at the beginning of my health journey, and Jesus transformed my life. Friend, this is where you find comfort in the promises of God's Word. Meditate on them day and night.

When fear and anxiety weigh you down, keep you isolated, and send you to your bed, pulling the covers over your head...grab your Bible. Trust me when I say, begin this discipline today. God's Word truly satisfies every craving in your heart. Be filled up like Jeremiah: "When your words came, I ate them; *they were my joy and my heart's delight*, for I bear Your name, O LORD God Almighty" (Jeremiah 15:16, emphasis mine).

4. **Practice gratitude.** Focus on the blessings in your life and thank God for them. When people observe how I eat (or see me not eating junk food), they sometimes speak negatively about my choices. For example, they'll say, "Oh, I forgot, you can't eat that." I love to turn this around and say, "I could eat that; however, I choose not to for my health. And I'm so grateful for the whole foods that I can eat. I don't feel deprived at all." My heart is full of praise and worship for the healing benefits of living this Sugar*Freed* life!

   First thing in the morning, during your quiet time with God, I recommend you write a gratitude list. Every day, you will find something to be thankful for as you gain victory in your weight-loss battle. Every day, choose joy—like this: "Be joyful always; pray continually; give thanks in all circumstances, for this is God's will for you in Christ Jesus" (1 Thessalonians 5:16–18).

5. **Take care of yourself.** This means your whole health—physically, emotionally, and spiritually. Get enough sleep, eat healthy, and exercise regularly to help manage stress and anxiety. Think back to our HEART transformation acronym. God calls us to care for our whole health and gives us practical ways to manage our heart health, which is the core—the wellspring of our livelihood.

   We can do everything on our Christian checklist: read the Bible, pray, attend church, and worship—yet God calls us to care for our whole health and gives us practical ways to do so. That's why you're reading this book! The Holy Spirit nudged you to take back control of your health. And that means caring for your body on God's path for you. He gives us instructions in His Word.

These daily biblical practices will anchor your day and keep anxiety at bay. Which of these practices do you need to implement?

I'm humming the song by Francesca Battistelli, "The Breakup Song." She's breaking up with fear. I broke up with fear and anxiety. Are you ready to break up with fear and anxiety?

Are you prepared for God to fan that flame in you as you redeem your walk by His Spirit? How will you face unexpected trials in the future? How will God call you to share your redemptive healing story? My heart overflows as I witness the women I have coached step up and step out into their calling with greater confidence to impact the kingdom of God! Expect the unexpected, my friend.

A Note to Your Former Self:

A Note to Your Future Self:

Transform-Action Task:

Chapter 15

Celebrating Freedom—
No Turning Back Now!

■ ■ ■

I warned you that this weight-loss battle is not for the faint of heart. Friend, I'm ready to wrap up this part of your journey and encourage you to keep in your heart that there is no turning back now. You are in this to win this. Gaining freedom and victory over your weight-loss battle is your ultimate goal. And now you have a plan.

Arm yourself with practical advice and success stories from myself and other women who have broken the *sugar shackles*—the chains of sugar and junk food addiction. Each of us ignited 24/7 fat-burning, and you can too!

And you now understand how highly addictive these hyper-palatable and cleverly marketed foods can be. They've caused a problem resulting in excess weight, but fortunately, it can be lost. You can reverse your metabolic chronic disease. You see the possibility in your future health and wellness. And I want to remind you, given the years of poor dietary advice, this is not all your fault. When I learned the science behind the SugarFreed lifestyle and discovered that it works, I finally let go of decades of guilt and shame. My condition was partially my fault, but God made a way out. Remember—it might not be our fault, but it is our job to fix it.

You also know this will be one of the hardest things you ever do emotionally, and you are ready to experience and push through all the feelings. Pause right now, and pick a positive emotion to push you to the next best choice for your health.

You commit this journey to Jesus. You know now that He guides you through His Word. You can join me in gratefulness over God's good smorgasbord of whole and healthy food to fuel our body, mind, and spirit. Your heart is open and ready for transformation in your relationship with food, feelings, and your heavenly Father! Join me in embracing this truth: *Food is fuel!*

I remember my decades of wandering through life as a *casual Christian*. I was trying my best to control all the things in my self-centered life. My weight, my finances, my children, my material possessions, my reputation, my career...I could go on, but you get the point. If I'm honest, I lived with a crushed heart but somehow managed to push through the pain. I showed up fake each day in my joyless life. Just going through the motions another day with my heart set on crawling back into bed and away from my exhausted life. Sigh.

Friend, I hope you feel hopeful in a life well lived. God has a beautiful way of turning things around when we dare to respond to the healthy conviction He lays on our hearts. I have written many words in these pages, but I will never have adequate words to express to the Father how grateful I am that He has forever changed my heart. The tremendous benefit of living a healthy lifestyle to point others to Jesus is beyond my wildest dreams.

Now I want you to remember: first and foremost, how and why God called you to turn things around with your health. And remember the truths of what I have shared with you in this entire book. Lessons on *hard, health, heart,* and *heavenly truths*! All those truths are a great way to summarize where we've been, where we are, and where we long to be.

I found the word *flourish* today in my quiet time. *Flourish.* I love that. I want that for you. God has that for you, too.

> But I am like an olive tree
> flourishing in the house of God;
> I trust in God's unfailing love
> for ever and ever.
> —Psalm 52:8

Imagine yourself flourishing in your short time on earth, feeling well, having more energy to face the day, and walking out the purpose God has for you. It's time to embrace and celebrate the freedom Christ offers you for your whole health. Like I always say, when you feel better, you serve better. Are you ready to respond?

Let's head back to the mountains for a few more stories. I climb mountains to embrace this newfound freedom and remind myself I'm never returning to my former ways of carrying so much extra weight on my body and shoulders. Yes. Remember my favorite mountain saying? *The mountains are calling, and I must go!* Join me.

Do you have a travel destination dream? A place on your bucket list? For decades, I only dreamed of visiting Ireland. I reasoned in my mind that, as an obese woman, I could never enjoy such an adventurous trip from the comfort of a car. I never wanted to spend the money and not be able to fully experience all that Ireland has to offer. It was just a dream in this Irish lassie's heart.

But God! Until the day I made that first choice and dedicated myself to taking back control. Once and for all. And God's mercy and grace kept me focused on this endeavor so that I would one day climb mountains.

Once I reached a healthy weight, the dream of visiting Ireland stirred in my heart, and it wouldn't let go. Let the planning begin! Where will you plan to go?

In Spring 2018 (after just five months of maintaining my new healthy weight), my daughter and I rented a car and went on the adventure of a lifetime—three weeks around the outer ring of Ireland's country roads. We hiked, biked, and climbed a mountain. To my surprise, we found a mountain to climb in the beautiful Glendalough National Park in County Wicklow.

As I read the park trail information, something sparked: "Pick the most challenging trail. You're ready!" And I did. I chose the White Trail, which would end up being an eleven-mile round-trip hike. Talk about hard!

That day, my pipe dreams materialized. Complete with blisters from my new hiking boots and an empty water bottle, I reached the summit of the White Trail. Tears of joy streamed while I stood on a summit I never dreamed possible. It was my most satisfying taste of success, of victory, in my battle over obesity and chronic disease. And it solidified my resolve and my heart's desire to celebrate this new and improved, abundant way of life.

I arrived at the celebration of a life lived by faith over my relationship with food. I am free. Sugar*Freed*.

God, in His goodness, moved so many mountains in my path to crave, choose, live, and be well for the glory of His good name. His good name is *Jehovah Rapha*. Healer.

My story doesn't end there on that summit of the White Trail in the beauty of Ireland. Because the Rocky Mountains of Colorado were calling me, too, *the mountains are calling, and I must go!* Come along with me. (Be sure to visit the Resources page for the link to some mountain victory scenes in the photo scrapbook.)

Returning to Colorado has been a blessing many times in recent years. I'll never forget those hidden tears on the side of that mountain path. God saw those tears and the sadness in my heart, and indeed, He did meet me on the side of that rocky path heading up to Nymph Lake. I'm filled with awe and wonder to this day in the way He showed up, pulled me up, and laid out my battle plan daily to one day, and now every day, walk in freedom from sugar and food addiction.

There are two more very memorable mountaintop moments I want to share with you before I go. In November 2022, I double-challenged myself with an extreme hike up the Manitou Incline in Manitou Springs, Colorado, and with a snowy climb up to Nymph Lake at the Bear Lake stop in Rocky Mountain National Park. I love, love, love to climb mountains now. Literally and figuratively, you will find me doing this every day.

"Kaitlin, there is no way I can climb that Manitou Incline. I'm old."

Well, my age was my excuse anyhow. If you are unfamiliar with this extreme hike, put the book down for a moment and look up Manitou Incline in Colorado.

This climb is a former supply line with 2,768 stair steps from former railroad ties. Yes, I said two-thousand-seven-hundred-sixty-eight stairsteps! Consider the stairs in a skyscraper. When was the last time you climbed up over one hundred floors? Woo! Even crazier, the climb is less than one mile, but the elevation change is 2,020 feet with an average grade of 41 percent and the steepest grade at 68 percent (now that's steep!).[45] It would *probably* require climbing some sections on your hands and feet—there was no *probably* about it, it did!

Just listen to my daughter's coercion, I mean convincing and cheer-leading…"Mom, you can do it! You'll love it. Think how you will feel when you get to the top!"

Challenge accepted. I imagined exactly how I would feel at the top of that climb. Exhilarated. Excited. Energetic! Well, maybe not that last one. That climb depleted my physical energy stores, but since it was the most extreme hike I've accomplished, it filled my heart with extreme emotions. I do my best to explain. Just trust me. That hike changed my life.

"I can do hard things. I can do really hard things. I can do really, really hard things!" And I can live to tell you about it. I choose to say this to you because you can do hard things by faith. With the power of God, His love, His grace and mercy, His purpose for your life … you can do the hard things. Oh, and let's not forget His gift of self-control. All those gifts of God fuel you to do the hard things.

When you do these hard things and begin to find victory in the small habit changes God puts on your heart for your health, you are highly motivated to cling with dear life to the momentum. Let this momentum, these gifts, and your change in heart lead to a transformation guaranteed to make you pinch yourself daily over the goodness of God. I do this every day. Pinch me, too, while I praise God for every mountain He's moved in my way for you to experience your healing breakthrough!

Speaking of praise, while in Colorado that November, I knew I needed to return to the scene of my turning point. We loaded into my cousin Jacque's car and drove toward Bear Lake in Rocky Mountain National Park.

The line to get into Bear Lake went for miles. On an ordinary adventure, we would've skipped it for a less crowded place in the park. But my daughter and dear cousin knew how important this day was to my story. To your story. I trust it will encourage you to face your mountain today.

When we finally exited the car, you would think I would've rushed to the Nymph Lake trail. It was the same trail I failed to climb with my husband. But nope, we did the easy hike first around Bear Lake. To be honest, I felt a little anxiety pop up about the Nymph Lake trail. What if I couldn't make it to the lake today? This nagging and negative self-talk shocked me after climbing the Manitou Incline just two days prior. However, I quickly took that thought captive and told myself to climb. There were no more condescending voices in my head like I had experienced at the lowest point in my life. Remember those imaginary hikers who tormented me as I sat exhausted on the side of that path?

"Look at the obese woman. No wonder she can't make it up this trail," chided Hiker A.

"If she had any self-control, she'd not be stuck sitting there like a bump on a log," judged Hiker B.

"Maybe she should get up and move her body. She needs more physical activity," shouted Boot Camp Hiker C.

No, no, no … you no longer have that control in my life!

"Let's go! Nymph Lake is calling my name!"

And we arrived. And I'll forever freeze the memory of this beautiful frozen lake in the beautiful Rocky Mountains in my mind. The best part? The climb was easy! Don't miss the photo in the scrapbook (see Resources page for the link).

Thinking back to the failed climb of 2015 just now, a new memory comes to mind as I write these words. I recall my husband saying to me when he came back down the trail, "You were so close!"

Pardon me while I get up and bawl for ten minutes.

Okay, I'm back. Yes, this truly just happened. I just sobbed and can now carry on.

"You. Were. So. Close."

You. Are. So. Close.

I knew wrapping up the words in this book would be hard. I knew there would be tears because my heart wants the same victory in Jesus for you. But wrapping this up, despite the cleansing tears, is cathartic. And it fills me with great hope for you.

I envision you running free in your newfound healthy lifestyle—vibrant, thriving, adventurous, climbing mountains, *made alive in Christ*!

During my quiet time this morning, I read more from Paul in Ephesians. It's a perfect prayer for you as we move toward the end of our time together.

For this reason I kneel before the Father, from whom his whole family in heaven and on earth derives its name. I pray that out of his glorious riches he may strengthen you with power through his Spirit in your inner being, so that Christ may *dwell in your hearts through faith*. And I pray that you, being rooted and established in love, may have power, together with all the saints, to grasp how wide and long and high and deep is the love of Christ, and to know this love that surpasses knowledge—that you may be filled to the measure of all the *fullness of God*. (Ephesians 3:14–19, emphases mine)

What a beautiful prayer. Paul eloquently addresses the Ephesians with many themes I want you to take away from your time in this book—*the heart*. God dwells right there in your heart through faith. We must rely on the faithfulness of God while deepening our faith (and don't forget, I have faith in you to do these hard things, too)—the fullness of God. Oh, friend, when we feel a hunger, a craving in our soul, I pray you will experience the fullness of God all day, every day.

God winked at me this morning before I sat in my cozy brown leather chair to share my heart with you. Today is the first anniversary of the day I conquered the Manitou Incline. How good is God that He gives us cherished memories? Even one year later, as I sit here with tears, He gives me a new lesson to pass along to you—a lesson about false summits.

As I huffed and puffed up that incline, I moved closer and closer to the point of victory. "At least I can see the end of this crazy adventure." Wrong. What I had in my sights for most of that hike was a false summit. "Are you kidding me?"

And that's life. Sometimes, we will be *so close* (as my husband assured me), only to find ourselves at the base of another mountain in our path. When we face a hard challenge like a weight-loss journey, there will be many ups and downs—guaranteed! Again, we must eat. But before you go, I must share a key passage from Hebrews again. I want you to reflect on your *hard, healthy, heart,* and *heavenly truths* through the lens of this call to action.

Therefore, since we are surrounded by such a great cloud of witnesses, let us throw off everything that hinders and the sin that so easily entangles, and *let us run with perseverance* the race marked out for us. Let us fix our eyes on Jesus, the author and perfecter of our faith, who *for the joy* set before him endured the cross, scorning its shame, and sat down at the right hand of the throne of God. Consider him who endured such opposition from sinful men, *so that you will not grow weary and lose heart.* (Hebrews 12:1–3, emphases mine)

The Hard Truth

Sin hinders us, and by nature, we are born this way. Our patterns and behaviors with food may weigh us down in body, mind, and spirit. Easily entangled. Ugh. As the author writes, *"Let us throw off everything…"* my flesh cries out, "But it's so hard! I must eat!" So, grab your journal, ask yourself a few questions, and answer honestly:

- When I indulge in food, does it lead to overindulgence?
- When I overindulge, can I identify the true source of this behavior? Is it heartbreak, loneliness, trauma, or fear of failure leading to another setback?
- Do I need to be comforted due to some intense feelings? Am I turning to food for that comfort? When did I last reach for the word of God instead of the refrigerator for comfort?
- Can I be content with what God asks me to do with my food choices?
- Are my food behaviors sinful?
- What is it that I truly crave?
- Am I addicted to sugar?

The Healthy Truth

I'm not a massive fan of running, so let's use this phrase, *"Let us run with perseverance the race marked out for us…"* metaphorically. At some point in your life, God will ask you to run. Continue in your journal with these questions:

- Will you run this race, your purpose for His glory, with perseverance? Or will you sit on the side of that mountain path gasping for air like I did in my morbid obesity, emotional immaturity, and spiritual apathy?

- Will you trade this apathy for action?
- What chronic health issues are you currently facing that require addressing?
- How hard will you run to reverse them?

The Heart Truth

Dear friend, if there is one lesson I'm passionate about for you to take away from this journey, it's the truth of your heart health. Again, this is not the heart health your cardiologist would concern himself with. It's the heart of this battle: the heart transformation leading to your destination. Your victory. We are here for the victory, right? This is why we should persevere while running the race called life.

God is cheering you on (as am I) to this victory and giving you all the tools and incentives you need to improve your heart health. He repeatedly reminds us of this in Scripture, like here: " ... *so that you will not grow weary and lose heart ...* "

I know, I understand that a weight-loss battle makes us weary. Trust me. And I know in hindsight that my victory and deliverance into freedom resulted from the true heart transformation. Now that I know what I know, I urge you to spend meaningful time on these questions and matters of the heart:

- How would I rate my heart health? Review the HEART acronym and respond to your emotions, thoughts, motivations, courage, and action.
- Do I need to evaluate my sins of omission (like gluttony and laziness)? Remember, sins of omission are a failure to act on what you *now* know.
- How am I filling up my heart daily? Do I prioritize quiet time with Jesus? Or am I filling the holes in my heart with comfort eating or Netflix binges while stuffing my face, non-stop social-media scrolling, and piling on more guilt and shame?

- Can I be *comfortable being uncomfortable* with what God has put on my heart for my health?

Tough questions, I know. Hang on to hope.

The Heavenly Truth

You do not need to answer these tricky questions alone. Yes, you have this problem, and it's time you fixed it, but you are never alone. Do not ever forget that.

As a Christ follower, you know this truth. You know it's time to face these hard truths. You know your excess weight is weighing you down in body, mind, and spirit, but you will work to improve your heart health because of your hope in Christ. I call this the *heavenly truth*! If God is for us, who can be against us? Besides, He has a seat for you, yes, *you and me*, at His table in the heavenly realms. Hallelujah! Can I get an amen?

Christ has done the heavy lifting for us. Check this out: "Let us fix our eyes on Jesus, the author and perfecter of our faith, who *for the joy* set before him endured the cross, scorning its shame, and sat down at the right hand of the throne of God!"

For the joy! For the joy set before Him, He endured the cross to rescue and free you. Oh, I could write a whole book about this. Christ sacrificed and surrendered His life on the cross for your joy. For my joy. This *freedom and greater joy* are for you when you fix your eyes on Jesus! For you to declare with me, *Hallelujah!* That is the truth of God's satisfying Word.

- Do you taste and see that the Lord is good?
- What action must you take daily to fix your eyes on Jesus?
- Jesus scorned the shame of the cross. What is God speaking to you about your guilt and shame?

I talk about hindsight a lot; we know it is 20/20. And because God dragged me through this journey and filled my heart with overflowing joy, it's my honor to share these heavenly truths with you—from the mountaintop, with a view. And you're invited to take in this scenery with me. Living a life of *freedom and greater joy* is meant for you.

So, there you have it: the whole truth and nothing but the truth. Well, at least I pray I've done this work of writing justice through these stories and practical application steps you can *act on* while contemplating the *hard, healthy, heart,* and *heavenly truths.*

It's time to wrap up these words, but I won't abandon you now! I would love nothing more than to continue to be your guide and your biggest cheerleader. Please grab my gift to you so we can connect and continue this conversation. The best place to start is with those soul cravings, so please enjoy the *Crush Your Cravings: The Ultimate Wellness Guide for Christian Women.* When you download this free guide, you will receive an invitation to join my free Facebook group for Christian women and receive my emails to encourage and exhort you. Visit the Resources page for the link.

I'll also introduce you to *The SugarFreed Me Weight-Loss Solution* program. My coaching tagline is *Holistic Health, Fueled by Faith*—a proven coaching program designed to help you bust your sugar cravings, promote weight loss, and live SugarFreed for life.

Don't wait—this is me calling you to take the next best step. Don't just think about doing it, *act!* The final step in the heart transformation —*act!*

I'm *acting* by covering you in prayer and leaving you with this final beautiful reminder from Scripture:

> *On this mountain* the LORD Almighty will prepare
> a feast of *rich food* for all peoples,
> a banquet of aged wine—
> the best of meats and the finest of wines.
> *On this mountain* he will destroy
> the shroud that enfolds all peoples,
> the sheet that covers all nations;
> he will swallow up death forever.
> The Sovereign LORD will wipe away the tears
> from all faces;

he will remove the disgrace of his people
from all the earth.
The LORD has spoken.
—Isaiah 25:6–8, emphases mine

WOW! What a feast that will be! I'm ready to move from the stump on the side of that mountain trail to a seat at this table in the heavenly realms. Are you ready to get up from the sidelines of life? Won't you join me?

Let's get fit in body, mind, and spirit and walk in the *freedom and greater joy* that Christ Jesus offers us today. I'll meet you on the mountaintop soon. You must see this view.

A Note to Your Former Self:

A Note to Your Future Self:

Transform-Action Task:

Acknowledgments

To my Lord and Savior, Jesus Christ, who planned this story of redemption and gifted me a healing story beyond my wildest dreams. In Psalm 40:1 (NIV), David testifies, "*I waited patiently for the Lord; he turned to me and heard my cry.*" But He did, indeed, wait patiently for me. He lifted me from the pit, set my feet on solid ground, and gave me a new song—a song of *freedom* and *greater joy* in pursuing His calling. Jesus, thank you.

I am grateful to my family for loving me through those many years of poor health. I see God's hand through the happy and hard, the thick and thin in all our circumstances. Thank you, Rob, for your unconditional love and support—especially when I shared that it was time to quit my full-time job. God was calling me into full-time service for Him. I love you immensely for accepting it was time for me to say, "Goodbye, Corporate America."

To Kyle, Kaitlin, and Mike, I wish I could have a do-over of many unhealthy choices, especially the food I put on the table. I trust your observation of my transformation will forever impact your future health. I love you all.

Special thanks to my literary agent, Debbie Alsdorf, and Books & Such Literary Agency for your belief in getting the message of Sugar*Freed* and health and wellness for God's glory into the world. This is just the beginning! A special shout-out to Jill Kemerer, my amazing project manager—thanks for keeping me on schedule!

To my editor and book cover designer, you jumped on this project when I needed you most and supported my dreams and desires for the book's vision. Thank you, Jennifer Edwards and Amber Weigand-Buckley. And my book launch manager, Karen Sargent! I am confident I'd be wandering around aimlessly without you all!

The call to share this message came at a high cost. Besides ditching a cushy corporate salary, I've invested heavily in business coaching to serve my clients and audience well. These women teach me many lessons about entrepreneurship, writing, and speaking. Every step I've taken, I've been blessed to learn from the best. Enormous thanks to Lori Kennedy and the team at *The Wellness Business Hub*, Judy Weber, Patricia Durgin, Anita Brooks (with the life-changing challenge to invest the *talents*), Suzanne Kuhn, Mary R. Snyder, Tammy Whitehurst, Lori Boruff, Linda Evans Shephard, the AWSA and SpeakUp communities, and Robyn Dykstra. And to my newest coach, Brielle Cotterman, and team. Thank you for believing in my vision of changing health and wellness for the glory of God.

Many friends sat in the muddy and miry pits with me over the years. David continues in Psalm 40:2, "*He lifted me out of the slimy pit, out of the mud and mire; he set my feet on a rock and gave me a firm place to stand.*" Those decades-long "*stand by me*" friends deserve special thanks for sitting in the lows and celebrating the highs with me. Lots of love to Dee-Dee Keefe, Theresa Hogan, Heidi Moyer, Jill Chafetz, and Dianne Larson for their years of cheers and drying my tears.

Thank you, Mom and Dad, for your love and laying a solid foundation and heritage of faith for me and my siblings. It made it easier to return to the "*solid rock*" David references in Psalm 40:2. I pray the impact continues for generations. Did you ever think I'd be a published author? Me, neither!

Profound thanks to my pastor, Adam Groh, for planting the seed with his passion for and preaching the word of God. He was right when he used to say, "First, it will be a daily discipline, and before long, it will be your delight!" I'm sure he'll be delighted to hear me say, "You were right!" I love my Bible! And where would he be without his lovely wife, Jenn—a dear friend! The church he faithfully shepherds is a loving, biblically-grounded, and supportive community I love calling home. Thank you to each of you who have prayed over and participated in spreading this project! I especially thank my Life Group friends, Jan, Maria, Sylvia, Diane, and Chris, for your prayers and party-planning skills.

Speaking of prayer, where would I be without my *PIT*? On the days I struggled to push through, my prayer intercessory team raised my arms to see me through. I appreciate your friendship, encouragement, exhortation, and prayers—Stacy Leicht, Missy Linkletter, and Cheryl Lutz. I love you girls!

To Olivia, for your listening ear and words of wisdom. You, no doubt, many times have kept me from slipping back into the miry pit!

This passion and project would be nothing if it weren't for the women I've had the honor to coach, guide, and have hard conversations with over coffee. Special thanks to the six women who were excited to share their weight-loss victories in the pages here to encourage others: Deborah Malone, Sara Schaffer, Heidi Moyer, Dee, Athena Dean Holtz, and Christina England. Your stories will change lives for the glory of God!

To every woman I've pushed (and sometimes pulled) toward honoring God with your body, mind, and spirit—I see you. I know where you've been, where you are, and where you long to be. And you are getting there! Keep chasing that victory because God has a big story and will use it through you. Don't just take my word for it; check out David's experience in Psalm 40:3, "*He put a new song in my mouth, a hymn of praise to our God. Many will see and fear the Lord and put their trust in him.*" Your story will change not just your life but many lives. Thank you for trusting me as your coach and confidante.

I'll end with one last verse from my favorite Psalm. I hope I didn't leave out one word of acknowledgment or one person involved in this project, and if I have, please forgive me. I have run out of words due to the goodness of God. It's too much to declare.

> Many, Lord my God,
> are the wonders you have done,
> the things you planned for us.
> None can compare with you;
> were I to speak and tell of your deeds,
> they would be too many to declare.
> —Psalm 40:5

Trusting the Lord will work wonders for you, too.
With Joy,
Christine Trimpe

SUGAR*freed*
Resources

SCAN ME

https://christinetrimpe.com/sugarfreed-resources/

Links To Christine's:

- SugarFreed grocery shopping list
- *Crush Your Cravings: The Ultimate Wellness Guide for Christian Women*
- Photo scrapbook of client success stories and mountain views

- Details about *The SugarFreed Me Weight-Loss Solution* program
- Spotify playlist
- Client testimony videos on YouTube
- Podcast interviews
- And Social Media links!

Notes

1   "Resolve," Merriam-Webster, accessed January 29, 2024, https://www.merriam-webster.com/dictionary/resolve.

2   "Quotations from John Muir," Sierra Club, accessed January 27, 2024, https://vault.sierraclub.org/john_muir_exhibit/writings/favorite_quotations.aspx.

3   "Psalm 121:1–2," BibleGateway, accessed August 6, 2024, https://www.biblegateway.com/passage/?search=Psalm+121%3A1%E2%80%932&version=NI.

4   *The Holy Bible, New International Version*® (Grand Rapid, MI: Zondervan Publishing, 1985), 790.

5   "Emotion," Merriam-Webster, accessed January 29, 2024, https://www.merriam-webster.com/dictionary/emotion.

6   "Thought," Merriam-Webster, accessed January 29, 2024, https://www.merriam-webster.com/dictionary/thought.

7   "Motivation," Merriam-Webster, accessed January 29, 2024, https://www.merriam-webster.com/dictionary/motivation.

8   "Courage," Merriam-Webster, accessed January 29, 2024, https://www.merriam-webster.com/dictionary/courage.

9   "Action," Merriam-Webster, accessed January 29, 2024, https://www.merriam-webster.com/dictionary/action.

10   "Craving," Dictionary.com, accessed January 24, 2024, https://www.dictionary.com/browse/craving.

11   "Physiological," Merriam-Webster, accessed January 29, 2024, https://www.merriam-webster.com/dictionary/physiological.

12   Jason Fung, MD, "The Blame for Fat Shaming," *The Fasting Method*, accessed January 29, 2024, https://blog.thefastingmethod.com/the-blame-for-fat-shaming/.

13   "What Is Intermittent Fasting?" DietDoctor.com, accessed January 29, 2024, https://youtu.be/VIhhrYjVhOk.

14   "Restore," Merriam-Webster, accessed January 29, 2024, https://www.merriam-webster.com/dictionary/restore.

15   "Adult BMI Calculator," Centers for Disease Control and Prevention, accessed January 29, 2024, https://www.cdc.gov/healthyweight/assessing/bmi/adult_bmi/english_bmi_calculator/bmi_calculator.html.

16 "Calculate Your Body Mass Index," National Institutes of Health, accessed January 29, 2024, https://www.nhlbi.nih.gov/health/educational/lose_wt/BMI/bmicalc.htm.

17 "What Is Metabolic Syndrome," National Institutes of Health, accessed January 29, 2024, https://www.nhlbi.nih.gov/health/metabolic-syndrome.

18 "What Is Metabolic Syndrome," National Institutes of Health, accessed January 29, 2024, https://www.nhlbi.nih.gov/health/metabolic-syndrome.

19 "Insulin Resistance and Prediabetes," National Institutes of Health, accessed January 29, 2024, https://www.niddk.nih.gov/health-information/diabetes/overview/what-is-diabetes/prediabetes-insulin-resistance.

20 "Hyperinsulinemia: An Early Indicator of Metabolic Dysfunction," National Institutes of Health, accessed January 24, 2024, https://www.ncbi.nlm.nih.gov/pmc/articles/PMC6735759/.

21 "Nonalcoholic Fatty Liver Disease (NAFLD) & NASH," National Institutes of Health, accessed January 29, 2024, https://www.niddk.nih.gov/health-information/liver-disease/nafld-nash.

22 "Motivation," Merriam-Webster, accessed January 30, 2024, https://www.merriam-webster.com/dictionary/motivation.

23 Miller, D. (Host). 2016–present. Business Made Simple [Audio podcast], https://building astorybrand.com/episode-37/.

24 Mel Robbins (@melrobbins), "Motivation is garbage. Stop waiting to feel like it. Whatever it is that you want - wake up and go get it. With hard work, patience and optimism - you can make," Twitter, May 20, 2022, https://twitter.com/melrobbins/status/1527689611413270530.

25 "Renew," Merriam-Webster, accessed January 30, 2024, https://www.merriam-webster.com/dictionary/renew.

26 "What is a Sin?" Southern Nazarene University, accessed January 30, 2024, https://home.snu.edu/~hculbert/sin.htm.

27 "Conscience," Dictionary.com, accessed January 30, 2024, https://www.dictionary.com/browse/conscience.

28 Matthew Henry Commentary on the Whole Bible (Concise), Romans 5, Bible Study Tools, accessed January 30, 2024, https://www.biblestudytools.com/commentaries/matthew-henry-concise/Romans/5.html.

29 "What is a Sin?" Southern Nazarene University, accessed January 30, 2024, https://home.snu.edu/~hculbert/sin.htm.

30 "3820.leb," Strong's Concordance, https://biblehub.com/strongs/hebrew/3820.htm, accessed January 30, 2024.

31 "Guilt," Merriam-Webster, accessed January 30, 2024, https://www.merriam-webster.com/dictionary/guilt.

32 "Shame," Merriam-Webster, accessed January 30, 2024, https://www.merriam-webster.com/dictionary/shame.

33 Kristi McLelland, *Jesus and Women: In the First Century and Now* (Nashville: Lifeway Press, 2022), 36.

34 Kristi McLelland, *Jesus and Women: In the First Century and Now* (Nashville: Lifeway Press, 2022), 37.

35 Kristi McLelland, *Jesus and Women: In the First Century and Now* (Nashville: Lifeway Press, 2022), 33.

36 Dr. Burk Parsons, "The Mortification of All Sins," *Tabletalk Magazine* 47, no. 5 (May 2023): 2.

37 Dr. Guy M. Richard, "Gluttony," *Tabletalk Magazine* 47, no. 5 (May 2023): 9.

38 Dr. Guy M. Richard, "Gluttony," *Tabletalk Magazine* 47, no. 5 (May 2023): 9.

39 Dr. Guy M. Richard, "Gluttony," *Tabletalk Magazine* 47, no. 5 (May 2023): 9.

40 Dr. Guy M. Richard, "Gluttony," *Tabletalk Magazine* 47, no. 5 (May 2023): 10.

41 Dr. Guy M. Richard, "Gluttony," *Tabletalk Magazine* 47, no. 5 (May 2023): 9.

42 "Redeem," Merriam-Webster, accessed January 27, 2024, https://www.merriam-webster.com/dictionary/redeem.

43 "Fear," Merriam-Webster, accessed January 31, 2024, https://www.merriam-webster.com/dictionary/fear.

44 "Self-control," Merriam-Webster, accessed January 31, 2024, https://www.merriam-webster.com/dictionary/self-control.

45 "Manitou Incline Facts," accessed January 31, 2024, https://manitousprings.org/where-to-play/manitou-incline/.

About the Author

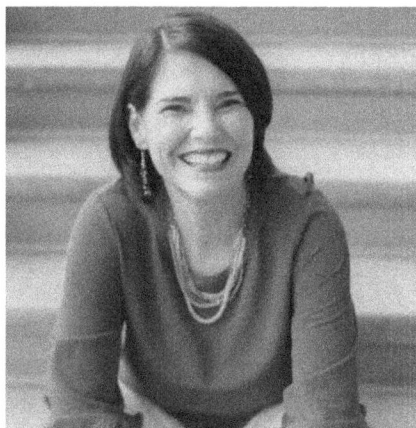

In a remarkable journey of faith and transformation, Christine Trimpe discovered a profound connection with Jesus that sparked a new purpose in her life. After decades as a *casual Christian*, she picked up her Bible, and Jesus changed her heart. This led to a one-hundred-pound weight loss and a complete lifestyle overhaul.

Christine's story resonates globally with readers, as published in publications like *Woman's World, First for Women*, and *Reader's Digest*. She has also earned a spot as a top success story on *DietDoctor.com*.

Certified as a Health and Wellness Coach through the American Association of Christian Counselors and a *SUGAR®* Licensed Practitioner, Christine now empowers women to quit sugar and claim weight-loss victory once and forever! As the founder of *The SugarFreed Me Weight-Loss Solution* program, her weight-loss program and community provide a path for women seeking both physical and spiritual fulfillment in a health and wellness journey.

Drawing from personal experiences, Christine encourages women to find joy amid life's challenges, emphasizing that God's Word satisfies every craving—mind, body, and spirit. She simply shares, "Ladies, you can do the hard things!"

When not developing transformative programs, Christine enjoys walking her grand pups, leading worship at her home church, and climbing mountains with her husband, Rob, and family. Learn more about her writing, speaking, and coaching at ChristineTrimpe.com and embark on a journey of freedom and greater joy with Jesus.

CONNECT WITH CHRISTINE

Thank you for reading Sugar*Freed*. Your support is so appreciated. Please leave an honest review on Amazon, Goodreads, and other platforms where books are sold. Your review will help other people on their journey to health and wellness freedom! Thank you in advance.

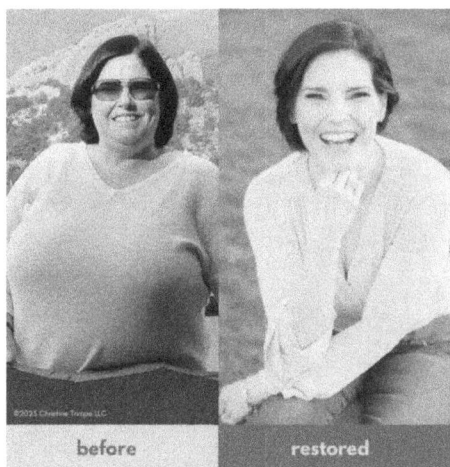

before   restored

All images used by permission and provided by: Before photo taken by the author. Restored photo taken by Sarah Wyatt-Stahl, You and Eye Photography, Berkley, Michigan

To invite Christine as a keynote speaker or teacher for your women's event, visit ChristineTrimpe.com/speaking/ or simply scan the QR code below.

SCAN ME

https://christinetrimpe.com/speaking/

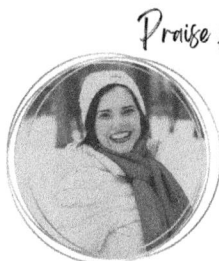

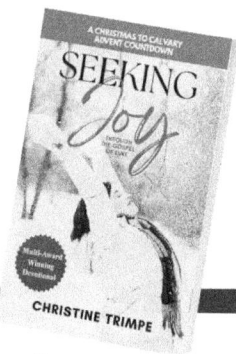